Take Charge of Your Life

101 WAYS

Enhance Your Self-esteem

TO STAY

Boost Your Metabolism with Mini-Meals

MOTIVATED

Don't Accept Not Trying

AND

Eat Healthier

LOSE WEIGHT

101 Inspirational quotes accompany each lifestyle enhancement

101 WAYS TO STAY MOTIVATED and LOSE WEIGHT

Donna Lynn

Founder of Donnacize Aerobics Inc. and Author of *Lose Your Stomach Forever The Donnacize Way*

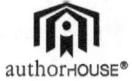

authorHOUSE®

AuthorHouse™ LLC
1663 Liberty Drive
Bloomington, IN 47403
www.authorhouse.com
Phone: 1-800-839-8640

Published by AuthorHouse   06/18/2014

ISBN: 978-1-4969-1902-1 (sc)
ISBN: 978-1-4969-1901-4 (e)

ACKNOWLEDGMENTS

I would like to express my deep appreciation and profound gratitude to my editor Tiara Carr for her enthusiasm, dedication and feedback. Thanks again Eric Cuffie for the images. To my son Tyrell, continue to be a light in the lives of the many children that you work with. Words cannot express the love that I have for you. To my nieces, nephews and godchildren, Patricia Cuffie-Jones, Derrick Cuffie, Tabitha Baxter, Winston Baxter Jr., Nicole Baxter, Kristina Baxter, William Baxter, Raven Baxter, Cynthia Baxter, Latika Diggs, Toni Chiarella and James Graves: this book is dedicated to all of you. Always know that if you put in the work, the results will come.

"Your crown has already been bought and paid for. All you have to do is put it on your head."

James Baldwin

Contents

PROLOGUE

Teachers often teach that which they love and want to learn more about themselves. I am no different. I wrote this book for my clients to benefit from, as well as to nourish my own desire to stay healthy in every dimension of life. My guess is that what has brought you to this book is exactly what has driven me to write it: the desire to make a drastic change in life, not only physically, but emotionally as well. I, too, want to remain motivated, eat an overall healthy, yet tasteful diet, and maintain a healthy weight; and this book is here to help us both.

Some of the life enhancements within this book derived from people just like you whose life experiences have taken them from one roller coaster ride to another as a result of poor diets, failed exercise plans and negative life experiences. Others developed from the valuable information I've read in books and articles, as well as what I've learned from seminars and daily conversations with friends, family members and colleagues.

Regardless of its origin, *101 Ways* is designed to motivate you in more ways than one. The goal is for you to make better life choices by living a healthy life filled with vitality and passion. These choices can be guided by the 101 tips listed herein, which I hope will provide you with greater insight, better understanding (of a healthy diet) and the motivation to move.

I want you to feel inspired and believe in the possibility of you being the best YOU ever. So, whether your overall goal is to get fit, search for a new career, or just enhance your life for the better, your first step is to take the initiative to change your mind-set and operate on a higher level. In order to do this, you must become mindful of your behaviors and thought patterns. When you are honest and open for change, change will happen. And this book will help you see that it does.

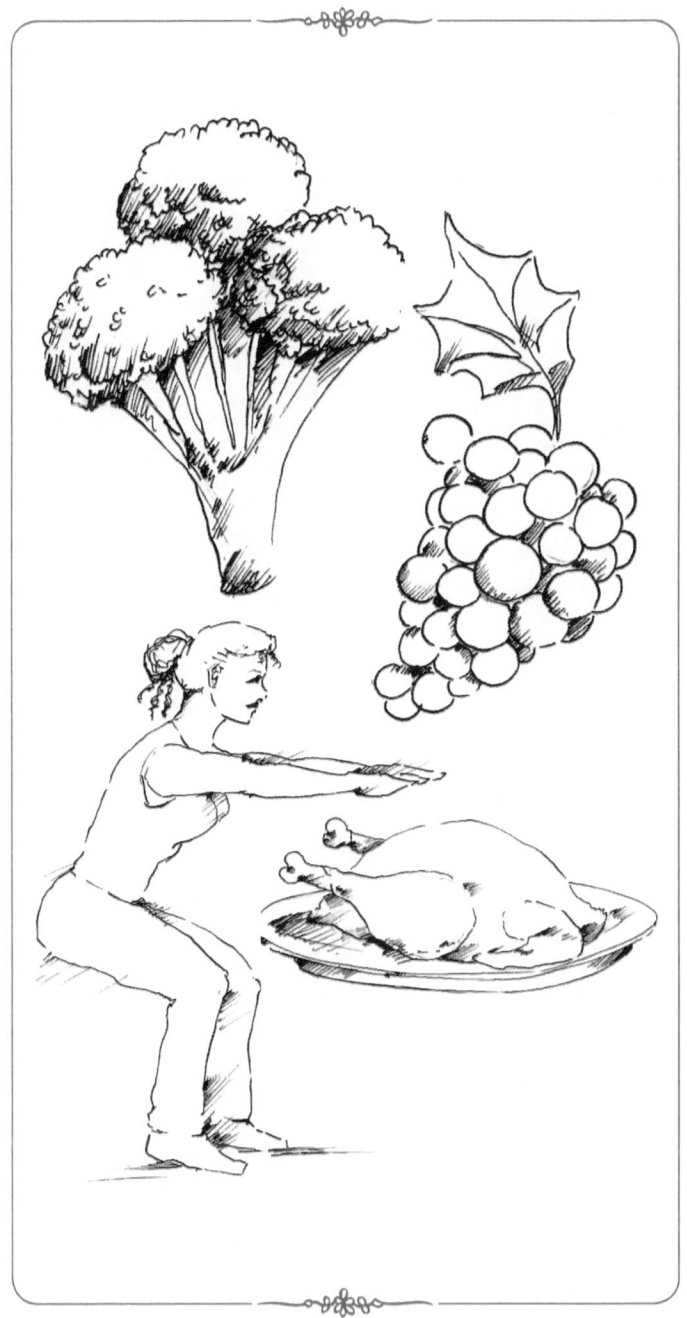

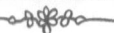

1. <u>You are Beautiful!</u>

Many people begin an exercise program in hopes of losing weight for an upcoming event — failing to realize that everyday is an event. Others want to lose weight because they simply don't like how they look compared to other people and want to look better. But since there is no one else like you, try not to compare yourself to others whom you perceive as prettier, richer, smarter, braver, or more together than you. This is a trap and a self-defeating cycle that you cannot win. Don't even compare yourself to who you used to be. No one is more beautiful than you are in this very moment! Don't focus on trying to be like anyone else. Just be who you are and know that you are beautiful no matter what.

"If you don't like something, change it. If you can't change it, change your attitude. Don't complain."

Maya Angelou

2. <u>Eat Your Last Meal at Least 4 Hours Before Bedtime</u>

When should I eat my last meal of the day? My clients have been asking me this question for many years and I'm pretty sure it will continue to be a question of interest for years to come. Depending on who you're quoting or asking, the answers may vary. Since I don't know of many studies which talk specifically about when to eat before bed when it comes to losing weight, I'm going to speak from my experiences and observations.

I exercise for a living, and I've had very busy days which led me to miss several meals. When this happened, I found myself eating late night dinners and falling fast asleep within an hour. I awakened feeling full, with heartburn and memories of a dream that was more intense than usual.

I've also observed my students who were trying to lose weight, and many times it was easy to distinguish my late night eaters from those who followed my 4-hour rule. My late night eaters had less energy and found it more difficult to lose weight. My 4-hour-rule followers had more energy throughout the day, moved with ease during class, and were more optimistic about their journey to good health.

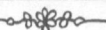

During late night hours, movement is at a minimum, so naturally, the body will *store* more calories than it will *burn*, and those stored calories become FAT. I believe you should make a conscious effort to keep your last meal portion-sized (see#42) and at a reasonable hour, while remembering to eliminate carbohydrates and fried foods. Some studies suggest that, *It doesn't matter when you eat, the question is what you're eating.* Although I believe this to be true to a degree, I also believe you should make an effort to evaluate your night eating and determine if you're eating based on boredom or emotion, rather than hunger. You can do this by establishing a set time for a nutritious dinner and not eating outside of that time. Your goal should be to separate suppertime from bedtime by at least 4-5 hours, so your food has a chance to digest. It takes about four hours for the average person's stomach to empty completely, so make your last meal one that will satisfy, yet not stuff you, and will aid in your healthy lifestyle.

> **"There are only two options regarding commitment. You're either in or you're out. There's no such thing as life in-between."**
>
> *Pat Riley*

3. <u>One Step Back? Two Steps Forward!</u>

No matter how many obstacles you run into, what matters most is that you're able to overcome each of them, one at a time. "Two steps forward, one step back" is a phrase often used negatively to describe someone who is having trouble making progress. But switched around, "one step back, two steps forward" means that although you may feel guilty about what you ate yesterday or how you haven't exercised in a week, you can still come out ahead by doing right today. A big mistake often made during the weight loss process is the uncertainty of not knowing how to get back on track when life throws a curve-ball. Many people experience feelings of hopelessness and believe that they need to start all over. Wrong! When missteps happen and send you one step back, a better strategy is to simply take two steps forward. You're still ahead of where you were before, and far beyond the starting line.

> *"Our greatest weakness lies in giving up.*
> *The most certain way to succeed is always*
> *to try just one more time."*
>
> *Thomas A. Edison*

4. <u>Drink 6-8 Glasses of Water per Day</u>

Your health is truly dependent on the quality and quantity of the water you drink. Dr. Fereydoon Batmanghelidj has spent most of his scientific life researching the link between pain and disease and chronic dehydration. His pioneering work shows that Unintentional Chronic Dehydration (UCD) contributes to, and even produces, pain and many degenerative diseases that can be prevented and treated by simply increasing water intake on a regular basis.

Your body needs water for vital functions like regulating body temperature, maintaining blood pressure, transporting nutrients, getting rid of wastes, and producing a huge variety of body fluids. Water lubricates your joints and also helps keep skin looking young, smooth and vibrant. An extra bonus is that it fills you up so you don't feel the need to eat as much throughout the day. If you are committed to a healthy lifestyle, make drinking enough water a habit in your life. It won't take long for you to feel the benefits, and it is a free investment for your long-term health.

"You're not sick; you're thirsty. Don't treat thirst with medication."

Dr. Fereydoon Batmanghelidj

5. <u>Walk Your Way to Great Health During Lunch</u>

The fundamental health benefits of walking during lunch are many — your metabolic system, weight, blood sugar, and cholesterol levels can all be strengthened while on the job. It is as simple as putting one foot in front of the other, yet as powerful and proven a therapy as customized diets and medications. Begin by eating a light lunch (without rushing) and walk the remaining minutes of your lunch break. Every minute of walking that you can fit into your day will increase your health and longevity. This exercise is low-impact, can be done almost anywhere, is easy on your muscles and joints AND you're still at work. The only things needed are comfortable walking shoes, a positive attitude and the willingness to get the most out of your eight-hour day. Research shows that you can attain a much higher level of conditioning and well-being if you actually train to improve your aerobic fitness by walking 30 minutes at least 4 days per week. Walking during lunch is the perfect compliment to a sensible diet that will help you to not only lose weight, but keep it off.

"Your life does not get better by chance, it gets better by change."

Unknown-Internet

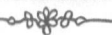

6. <u>Exercise to Help Reduce Low Back Pain</u>

Studies show that low back pain is the most common disability for persons under the age of 45, and is often caused by overuse of back muscles, and muscle strain or injury. During a lifetime, low back pain will affect 60-80% of American adults. According to some sources, it is estimated that up to 50% of U.S. adults will have low back pain symptoms within any given year. Although the causes of most low back pain vary, the best way to reduce the effect is to exercise. Exercising on a regular basis helps you learn how to protect your back so that you'll stay mobile and comfortable as you age. In most individuals, pain stems from an injury after lifting a heavy object or from making an abrupt movement. A regular exercise program can improve your flexibility, help you learn how to lift properly, and protect you from pain by improving and strengthening your core muscles. A balanced workout of back, abdominal, stretching and strengthening exercises combined with low impact aerobics will help reduce low back pain.

"The pain of today, is the victory of tomorrow."

Unknown-Internet

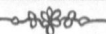

7.   <u>Exercise 3-4 Days Per Week</u>

Physical activity is any body movement carried out by the skeletal muscles that requires energy. When you perform any type of physical activity 3-4 days per week, you are burning calories, taking control of your body, and becoming healthier and stronger. Thirty to forty-five minutes of aerobic exercise, at least three times per week, will strengthen and condition the heart muscle, control your weight and blood pressure, and reduce your risk of heart disease. This process speeds up your metabolism so your body is conditioned to burn fat more quickly than the average non-exerciser. Be sure to check with your health care provider before beginning any exercise program. (Complete the Physical Activity History Questionnaire in the back of the book, Appendix B).

> *"Losing weight is hard. Maintaining weight is hard. Staying overweight is hard. Choose your hard."*
>
> *Unknown- Internet*

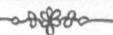

8. Practice Good Postural Habits at All Times

Good posture says a lot about a person, as it influences not only how your body feels, but also how you feel about your body. Good posture is the position of the parts of your body in relation to each other. When you practice sound posture, your waist can become smaller, your confidence can become greater and your weight can become balanced and efficient. For example, when standing, your head, shoulders, and hips should line up, one comfortably above the other. When sitting, be sure that your back is aligned against the back of the chair and your feet are comfortably flat on the floor. Avoid slouching or leaning forward, even when you grow tired from sitting in the office chair for long periods of time. Don't neglect your posture. It can make a great impact on your overall health.

> *"Just believe in yourself, even if you don't, pretend that you do and at some point you will."*
>
> *Venus Williams*

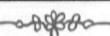

9. <u>Leave the White Breads Alone</u>

You needn't dread bread in general; however, you may want to focus on certain types of bread. Dark whole grain breads can provide a natural source of fiber and complex carbohydrates. In addition, studies show that some breads actually reduce the appetite. Researchers found that students who ate 12 slices a day of dark, high fiber bread (with no additives) felt less hunger on a daily basis and lost an average of five pounds in two months. Others, who ate white bread, were hungrier, ate more fattening foods and lost no weight during that same period.

One slice of commercially prepared white bread contains 80 calories, according to the U.S. Department of Agriculture's National Nutrient Database. The average slice of whole grain bread contains only 60-70 calories, is rich in complex carbohydrates and delivers a surprising amount of protein. The key is to eat dark, rich, high-fiber breads such as pumpernickel, whole wheat, mixed grain, oatmeal, etc.

> *"The healthy man is the thin man. But you don't need to go hungry for it: Remove the flours, starches and sugars; that's all."*
>
> *Samael Aun Weor*

10. <u>Don't Drink Your Calories</u>

"You may be surprised at the number of calories you drink in a day," say researchers from the American Institute for Cancer Research. Their survey found that about 20 percent of the average adult's daily caloric intake comes in liquid form. Research shows that our brains don't "register" calories in liquid form, making them particularly easy to overlook. Sodas are by far the biggest source of sugar in the average American's diet, with 40 grams of sugar per 12 ounces. And most of the calories from soft drinks, sweet teas and gourmet drinks add up to big weight gains over time. If you cut back or cut out the sodas, then you're cutting out a lot of calories. Champagne, wine, mixed drinks, spiked eggnog and other alcoholic beverages are also heavy on calories and light on nutrients. Even non alchoholic drinks like hot chocolate and plain egg nog can supply hundreds of calories. When you are thirsty, try drinking water, diluted juice, soy milk or green tea.

> *"Motivation is what gets you started. Habit is what keeps you going."*
>
> *Unknown-Internet*

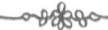

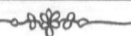

11. <u>Don't Count Failures</u>

The old saying, "If at first you don't succeed, try, try again" is true. The more times you try to accomplish something, the more likely you are to actually do it. So, what if your last attempt failed? Tell yourself, "Okay, that was just one of five or twelve attempts or however many it will take." It doesn't matter how many times you failed, the next time could be the one. So don't count failures — count successes, and never stop trying.

> *"I've missed more than 9000 shots in my career. I've lost almost 300 games. Twenty-six times I've been trusted to take the game winning shot and missed. I've failed over and over and over again in my life. And that is why I succeed."*
>
> *Michael Jordan*

12. <u>Exercise for Menopause Symptom Relief</u>

Many of the women I've spoken with have stated that a regular exercise regime has helped relieve *some* of their menopause symptoms. Menopause, or "the change," is a normal stage in every woman's life, usually occurring after age 45, that can bring uncomfortable and sometimes lasting effects on the body. Hormonal changes in a woman's body manifest as physical symptoms that include night sweats, "hot flashes," moodiness, sadness, irritability and sleeplessness. Exercise can play a key role in making the transition through menopause easier, as it enhances health, happiness and productivity during the second half of life. A Pennsylvania study found that being physically active does not necessarily *cure* menopause, but it does help postmenopausal women cope with stress, anxiety and depression. Exercise not only has the ability to decrease menopausal symptoms, but it allows more and more women the opportunity to live an overall healthy lifestyle because of it.

> *"Women are always being tested...but ultimately, each of us has to define who we are individually and do the very best job we can to grow into it."*
>
> *Hillary Clinton*

13. Eat Breakfast Daily

Breakfast is the first and most important meal of the day. It means we "break the fast" of not eating overnight to begin the new day. The most

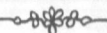
common reason cited for the value of breakfast comes from several large studies that have shown breakfast eaters to be thinner and healthier than breakfast skippers. A healthy breakfast provides the first fuel of the day for our bodies, giving us a sustained release of energy (calories) which aids to delay the symptoms of hunger for several hours. Our bodies work all through the night repairing and healing, so when we wake up in the morning it needs food for energy. A growing body of evidence suggests that a breakfast rich in protein and fiber can have a significant impact on the appetite and number of calories eaten throughout the day. An unhealthy breakfast filled with sugary foods can cause a quick spike in blood sugar and energy, but soon thereafter, both blood sugar and energy decline rapidly, bringing on hunger. Remember, it doesn't have to be much. In fact, a light breakfast of just a couple hundred good calories will do the trick.

> *"The first wealth is health."*
>
> *Robert Waldo Emerson*

14. Enhance Your Self-Efficacy

Self-efficacy refers to your belief in your ability to successfully take action and perform a specific behavior or task. When you start

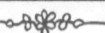

thinking about changing a health habit, a big factor in your eventual success is whether you have confidence in yourself and your ability to change. Setbacks will happen, but a single setback should not be the reason to abandon all of your good efforts. Enhance your self-efficacy by pushing through and successfully completing your goals no matter what.

Sometimes a wrench is thrown into your healthy lifestyle attempt unexpectedly and you're thrown off your routine and back into your old pattern or behavior. The temptation is to say, "What the heck, I might as well write off the whole week or month." Instead, try forgiving yourself and moving forward. Sticking to a strict exercise and eating plan 24/7 is not the easiest task to conquer on the first try. It can also be unrealistic and a formula for failure. The next time you have a set back, don't beat yourself up; instead, forgive yourself, forget it, and move on! The beautiful thing about life is that you're blessed with another day to try it again. Don't waste the experience by complaining and not fully enjoying the process. Enhance your self-efficacy and move forward. (Complete the Self-Efficacy Scale in the back of the book, Appendix C).

> *"The world of achievement has always belonged to the optimist."*
>
> *Harold Wilkins*

15. <u>Boost Your Metabolism with Mini-Meals</u>

Your metabolism is the rate at which your body burns calories to sustain life. A faster metabolism will let you eat more calories each day without gaining significant weight. Studies show that mini-meals, spaced 3-4 hours apart, not only keep blood sugar levels steady, but also increase metabolism, and are much better for you than 2 or 3 heavier meals per day. The mini-meal practice encourages your body to boost its metabolic rate rather than slow it down. Remember: we're talking about *light* meals — just two or three-hundred calories at a time that include a balance of proteins and carbohydrates. For example, turkey, chicken breast, yogurt and nuts are high in protein and should be included in the mini-meal plan. You also want to focus on foods in their natural state (complex carbohydrates) like vegetables, whole grains, and brown rice, as they keep your brain working at optimal levels throughout the day. By eating a moderate portion of complex carbohydrates every 3-4 hours, you keep your energy level steady. Small meals throughout the day also help control cravings, prevent overeating, and help you to stay ahead of the glucose curve which causes cravings.

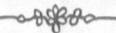

> *"Take pride in how far you have come and have faith in how far you can go."*
>
> *Internet-Unknown*

16. Don't Procrastinate

"I'll lose weight after the holidays," "I'll start eating healthier next week," "I'm too broke to go to the fitness club," "I'm too stressed," or "It's just not the right time." People come up with all sorts of reasons why now, today, just isn't the right time to complete a task, work on a project or change their lives. That's because procrastination is a deeply ingrained pattern of behavior that allows people to set up artificial barriers to put off what they can do today. When procrastination is practiced on any task, for any length of time, stress and anxiety are sure to follow. The key to controlling this destructive habit is to first recognize when the procrastination begins, understand why it happens (even to the best of us), and then take active steps to manage your time and outcomes better. You may also want to try breaking your goal into manageable, bite-sized steps. The bigger your goal or change, the more quickly it can send you into an overwhelmed state. Of course, you won't break the habit of procrastination overnight, but managing this habit may be the single most positive action you can make to improve the quality of your life.

> *"Marathon runners don't worry about the conditions, they just run anyway."*
>
> *Unknown-Internet*

17. <u>Pick a Time to Exercise and Stick with It</u>

There's just no easy way around it — if you want to achieve your fitness goals, you *have* to stay committed. That's why you must pick a time to exercise and stick with it. This way, when something comes up (and it will), you already know that you have a prior commitment (your exercise regime) that you cannot change or cancel. When you choose a specific time to exercise, you should fight for that time and let nothing get in your way. Everything else can come before or after your scheduled exercise time, but not during! Your exercise is your commitment to yourself, so stick with it.

> *"What you get by achieving your goals is not as important as what you become by achieving your goals."*
>
> *Henry David Thoreau*

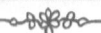

18. <u>Don't Accept Not Trying</u>

I borrowed this from basketball great Michael Jordan: "Know what you want and focus on getting there. As long as you do your best, you'll have accomplishments along the way, but you absolutely CANNOT ACCEPT NOT TRYING." For me, when self-doubt creeps in and I question whether the time and effort I'm spending on a project is worth it, I remind myself that if I keep taking action, reviewing my feedback, making adjustments and repeating the process over, I will achieve my goal. You, too, have the power to do something that will get you closer to your healthy weight and dietary goals. Choose something to change today, stick with it, and DON'T ACCEPT NOT TRYING!

> *"It's not whether you get knocked down; it's whether you get up."*
>
> *Vince Lombardi*

19. <u>Eat Soup Daily</u>

This simple dietary change will have you shedding pounds in no time: eat a bowl of soup at least once a day in place of one of your meals. Nutritious, low-salt soups are especially beneficial, as they fill you up and flush waste from your body. Part of the satisfaction you get from having broth-based soup is that you can eat a large portion while still sparing calories. Your mouth likes the extra food, your brain is turned on by knowing you're having more, and your stomach stays full longer. Add a glass of water, wheat or no-salt crackers and a piece of fruit, and you've just shed several inches from your waistline. This healthy meal once or twice a day will have you shedding pounds faster than ever. Go for homemade soups instead of cream or canned soups whenever possible, as they are loaded with salt and additives. You can also replace sugary snacks with a bowl of soup in between meals to help control your hunger.

> *"Both belly bulge and love handles are about excess body fat, not lack of muscle. Crunches and ab exercises are, therefore, not the solution. The best way to reduce these problem areas is to reduce your overall body fat percentage, and we all know that that requires diet and exercise."*
>
> *Jillian Michaels*

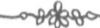

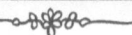

20. <u>Become a Fruit-Anista</u>

In order to become a fruit-anista you must first start by eating more fruit; it's the easiest way to get away with snacking on something sweet without jeopardizing your diet. If you already love fruit but just want more variety, try these delicious alternatives that also offer amazing health benefits: Instead of the everyday apple, try a papaya. A medium papaya has even more fiber than a medium sized apple. If you eat bananas for their dietary benefits, a kiwi is another good source of potassium. Watermelon and Guava are both rich in lycopene, the red pigment that's linked to a lower risk of cancer and heart disease. Instead of an orange, star fruit may be a more exciting alternative. It's a little sweet, a little acidic, is similar in nutrition, and offers a healthy dose of vitamin C, as well as choline for healthy cells. Remember — the more varied your diet, the more likely you are to get all the vitamins and essential minerals you need, as well as phytonutrients (a substance believed to be beneficial to human health that helps prevent various diseases).

> *"We can make a commitment to promote vegetables and fruits and whole grains on every part of every menu. We can make portion sizes smaller and emphasize quality over quantity. And we can help create a culture — imagine this — where our kids ask for healthy options instead of resisting them."*
>
> Michelle Obama

21. Get the Entire Family Involved

Talk with your family about your fitness goals and how important fitness is to your health. From an early age, children model themselves after what their parents do — not what they say. Next time you head to a store close by, walk instead of driving, and take the kids with you. Children are becoming less active and family fitness time is almost non-existent. You can play the important role of making sure that you and your family are active by taking the first step and moving daily. Family exercise will improve the health of you and your loved ones, develop stronger relationships amongst all of you, and make exercise more fun.

Not only do healthy activities bring families closer together, they also help decrease the risk of developing other disorders such as type 2 diabetes, obesity and cholesterol abnormalities. In fact, obesity has become the most prevalent chronic health problem for families and is one of the easiest to combat. So, increase the overall condition of yourself and your loved ones — body and mind — by becoming the physically fit model for your family. It's a gift that lasts a lifetime.

> *"For every minute you spend debating whether or not to work out, you could be working out."*
>
> *Unknown-Internet*

22. <u>Visualize</u>

When it comes to visualizing your weight loss: See it, Feel it and Enjoy it. For instance, if your goal is to fit back into your college attire, move the clothes that are now too small or too snug to the forefront of your closet and visualize yourself fitting into them again. If you could fit into them before, you can fit into them again.

So what is the right way to visualize what you want? Do you visualize each exercise you plan to do? Do you visualize your diet before you actually start it? No. You can start by visualizing your *end result*. Research has shown that the most effective way to visualize your end result is to do a present reality check right after visualizing your desired future. If losing weight is your goal, you must first visualize your ideal body weight realistically. The reality check keeps your vision real and prevents your goals from turning into farfetched dreams. The ability to hit a goal is limited only by your imagination and how effectively you visualize hitting that target. Use positive visualization to help reach your goals while enjoying all of your accomplishments along the way. Remember: As you visualize your goals, you must take action. Visualization with no action will keep you in the same size.

> *"He who has health, has hope. And he who has hope, has everything."*
>
> *Arabian proverb*

23. Love Yourself First

You will feel loved and lovable when you feed yourself healthy food, and get consistent exercise and sleep. When you ignore your health, you are sending yourself the message that you are not worth loving even from yourself. When you love self, your health becomes important and you exist in a strong package you're proud of.

Love yourself for who you are and don't try to become someone else; only strive to be a better you. Some consider loving one's self negative or arrogant behavior, but it isn't. Loving yourself is like loving someone else you deeply care about. But instead of giving that love and attention to another person, you give it to yourself by exercising and incorporating healthy foods into your diet.

"I know where I'm going and I know the truth, and I don't have to be what you want me to be. I'm free to be what I want."

Muhammad Ali

24. <u>Be Realistic</u>

How many times have you started the new year with an unrealistic resolution, only to find yourself weeks later frustrated and disappointed? The best way to avoid disappointment is to learn how to set realistic and attainable goals. If you want to begin your lifestyle change during the summer, a good approach may be to set a goal such as, "By *next* summer 1 will be 20-50 pounds lighter." Losing weight is a lifestyle choice that takes time. Often, dieters set up "no-win" situations for themselves by having unrealistic expectations about how much weight they can lose in a certain amount of time. But keep in mind how long it took you to put on the extra pounds and how long it's been since you've been physically active. These questions are important, as they will play a major role in your success, and they form the foundation of how you approach your plan. Repeatedly failing to stick to your goals means that either your goal is out of reach or that you haven't quite figured out *how* to reach it. Don't add unnecessary stress to your life by setting unrealistic goals. Be realistic and enjoy the process.

"Your attitude determines your altitude!"

Denis Waitley

25. Set Short-Term Goals

The best way to succeed is to set realistic short-term goals. Your end result may be to lose 70 pounds, but your present focus should be on losing the first five. When you accomplish short-term goals, your momentum is heightened and you're more excited to move to the next level. Don't make the mistake of sabotaging yourself because the end result doesn't come as swiftly as you would like. The best time of your life is now, so set short-term goals and keep moving towards the big finish.

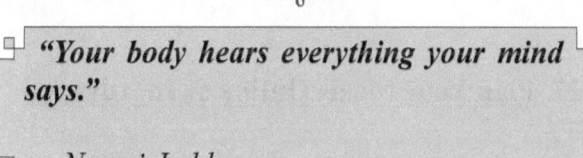

"Your body hears everything your mind says."

Naomi Judd

26. <u>Join an Aerobics Class</u>

Joining an aerobics class is a fun way to get fit, especially if you don't like exercising alone. These classes are designed to target the cardiovascular system and get participants involved and moving for at least 45 minutes. Participants often form relationships that allow them to motivate and encourage one another while in class and aerobic instructors usually give participants the option to do movements at a low or high intensity. The level of intensity is determined by how high you raise your arms and lift your legs — not by how fast or slow-paced the exercises are. Cardiovascular fitness is an ongoing process and requires consistent reinforcement. To maintain a level of fitness that will produce positive results, try doing aerobic exercises at least three times per week.

"To maximize fat burning, exercise the body before you feed it."

Unknown-Internet

27. <u>Plan Your Meals Online or In Advance</u>

Developing a meal plan will help you eat a more nutritious, well-balanced diet that includes nutrient-rich foods from each of the five food groups. You can even use a meal planner, just like a day planner, to help you keep track of your meals. This can be a formal printed or interactive planner, or simply a few notes jotted down on the back of an envelope. With a little preparation, planning your meals online or in advance can help you save time and money at the grocery store. Nielsen research indicates that meal planning is "one of the largest and fastest growing online activities." To assist consumers, retailers have responded with iPhone and Android smartphone applications that assist with meal planning. When used properly, these applications help users stay focused and in control of what they're eating. When you plan your meal ahead of time, you may be more inclined to purchase healtheir foods and pack them to-go with you. This results in saving you money, saving your health, and creating a meal specific to what you want each day. You may also find that you can better manage your weight when you plan and prepare meals at home more often.

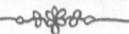

> **"Those who have no time for healthy eating will sooner or later have to find time for illness."**
>
> *Edward Stanley*

28. Laugh

Laughing helps us to keep a sense of perspective and can play an important role in defeating stress or depression. When you experience humor, distressing emotions actually dissolve. Laughing stimulates the immune system and has the power to suppress illnesses, depression and painful feelings. Have you heard the old saying, "Laughter is the best medicine"? Well, it's true! Read something humorous, visit a comedy club or watch a funny movie. When you laugh heartily, you're actually massaging your heart, lungs and digestive system. We know that exercising and eating low-fat meals will reduce the risk of heart disease, but maybe one day exercise, a healthy diet, and *laughing*, will be documented as the key to a healthy and prosperous lifestyle.

"I laugh at myself. I don't take myself completely seriously. I think that's another quality that people have to hold on to...you have to laugh, especially at yourself."

Madonna

29. "X" Your Calendar When You Exercise

Marking your calendar on the days you exercise helps to keep you focused, as it prevents you from getting out of your routine. If you've had a hard time motivating yourself to exercise, try this simple, yet powerful practice. Keep a pocket calendar with you, or hang one up at home or work, and mark every time you exercise. This habit serves as a constant reminder of the number of days you exercised in a week, month and year. If several days are missed, it is an instant cue for you to get back on track. You can mark an "X" on the day you exercised, add a set time to exercise, and include the type of activity. Write in ink — not pencil — and don't let anything interfere with your scheduled appointment! When three consecutive days are unmarked, stop what you're doing and include exercise onto your calendar immediately.

> *"You have to do what others won't to achieve what others don't."*
>
> *Unknown-Internet*

30. <u>Exercise with Your Significant Other</u>

If motivation (or lack thereof) keeps derailing you from the fitness track, a workout partner may be just the boost you need to get — and stay — in shape. When you begin an exercise program with your significant other, it may help you to exercise longer and more consistently than if you did it alone. If you both are motivated by different types of physical activity, change it up. Try your partner's exercise ideas one day, and then yours the next. If you have trouble agreeing — compromise. Be open-minded, and keep your partner's needs (fitness level, goals, comfort level) in mind too. For many couples, one partner tends to favor cardio (typically women) while the other tends to favor strength training (typically men). By working out together you can balance your workout program to include more of both. In addition, my clients found that the new bond they'd established through mutual exercise, had actually improved their relationships in other ways too. A large number said that working out with their partners improved their sex lives,

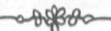

allowed them to achieve their exercise goals and helped them to stay focused.

> *"When we try to exercise alone, we can feel isolated and uninspired; together we can achieve our fitness goals."*
>
> *Felicity Luckey*

31. <u>Reduce the Stress in Your Life</u>

Stress management starts with identifying the sources of stress in your life. Unfortunately, this isn't always as easy as it sounds. Stress is the body's physical, mental, and chemical reaction to circumstances that frighten, excite, confuse, endanger or irritate us. Sometimes your true sources of stress aren't always so obvious, and it's all too easy to overlook your own stress-inducing thoughts, feelings, and behaviors. Sure, you may know that you're constantly worried about work deadlines. But maybe it's your procrastination, rather than the actual job demands, that leads to deadline stress. Constant pressure to meet the needs of family, employers, friends and self can be overwhelming. Even worse, stress can lower your immune system, leading to illness, and stress can lead to rash decision-making.

When you are mentally and physically strong, your body is better able to withstand the stressors of life. An exercise routine that gets your heart pounding for at least 30 minutes releases the "feel good" brain chemicals that reduce stress and depression. Laughter, music, yoga and meditation are also excellent sources of natural stress relief that can help you release, relax and rejuvenate for a lifetime.

> *"Time and health are two precious assets that we don't recognize and appreciate until they have depleted."*
>
> *Denis Waitley*

32. Exercise While Watching Television

After a long day at work or at home taking care of the family, most adults want to sit down in front of a television to unwind. Statistics show that the average American watches at least three hours of television per day. For some people, that may seem like a lot of time, but for others it's pretty normal. What would you say if I told you that you can continue to relax in front of the TV, and also fit in some exercise? There is a commercial of at least 3 minutes every 15-30 minutes when you are watching normal TV. This is the perfect opportunity to fit in a

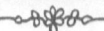

mini-workout. It is recommended that adults amass 30 minutes of moderate intensity exercise at least 3-4 days per week. If you get moving during the commercial breaks, you can easily meet those recommendations. Just think, you can meet or even surpass the recommendations easily while still sitting in front of the television.

You can start by stretching — sit on the floor with your legs apart and reach for your toes. Ready to do more than stretch? Try strengthening your abdominal muscles during commercial breaks. For example, you can lie on your back and bend your knees with your feet still on the floor and your hands crossed on your chest. Place your feet beneath the sofa for support, or have a family member hold them down for you. Exhale as you lift your back as high as you can and inhale going back down. Complete as many sit-ups as you can within 60 seconds. While you're on the floor you can also lie on your side and perform leg lifts that tighten and firm your gluteus maximus and quadriceps muscle groups, all while viewing your favorite program. Don't feel like getting on the floor? Try performing standing knee lifts and basic squats. It's very easy to sit in front of the television for hours, but do your body a favor and move a little at least one of those hours. What else do you have to lose... but weight?

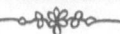

> **"Be miserable. Or motivate yourself. Whatever has to be done, it's always your choice."**
>
> *Wayne Dyer*

33. <u>Keep the Benefits in Mind</u>

The positive benefits achieved from regular exercise include, but are not limited to:

    a. Reduced risk of heart disease, high blood pressure, and diabetes
    b. Reduced risk of colon cancer
    c. Healthy and strong bones
    d. Less chance of catching colds and flu
    e. Better weight management
    f. Increased energy
    g. Better sleep
    h. Less anxiety and depression
    i. Enhanced self-esteem

Studies have consistently found that physical activity reduces the risk of cardiovascular disease. That is, those who perform moderate amounts of activity or those who are moderately fit have the lowest risk. Try being active 30 minutes or more each day. If you're unable to get the 30 minutes in all at once, try getting them in short increments.

> **"Physical fitness is not only one of the most important keys to a healthy body, it is the basis of dynamic and creative intellectual activity."**
>
> *President John F. Kennedy*

34. <u>Hire a Personal Trainer</u>

If you have difficulty finding the motivation to exercise alone, a personal trainer may be just what you need to get started. A personal trainer can create a customized program to suit your specific goals and lifestyle. They can ensure that you stay motivated and excited about the process and can even meet you at a location that's convenient for you. A skilled trainer will assess your specific needs, injuries, health conditions or training goals (maybe that 10 kilometer race you're dreaming about, for example). The trainer can then develop a personalized plan with clear timelines and short-term achievement goals that will safely and effectively enable you to succeed. Occassionally, we run into plateaus during our fitness progression. Those are normal. A personal rainer is trained to help you to push past those hurdles and move on to the next step. Your personal fitness trainer will always be there, just waiting for you to show up. It's much more difficult to put off going to the gym when someone is expecting you! Plus, your trainer reminds you of your reasons for wanting to exercise, and helps you understand why it's so important even when you feel as though you could talk yourself out of it. He or she is there to support you as you work towards enhancing the quality of your life now and in the future. Let your trainer guide you and teach you how to be your own personal trainer!

> *"You've got to say, 'I think that if I keep working at this and want it badly enough I can have it.' It's called perseverance."*
>
> *Lee Iacocca*

35. Aim for Balance

Most women aren't just walking a tightrope these days, they're doing cartwheels and backflips and still managing to stay in control of their busy lives. If you are working a 40-hour work week and raising a family, finding time for yourself can be a task. A way to aim for balance could include freeing yourself of certain responsibilities, cutting out extra activities, or delegating tasks to others. Make it easier on yourself, not harder. If your life lacks balance, don't get frustrated and don't neglect your health. Rather, think of a balanced life as a smooth juggling act. Just remember: if you're trying to catch too many balls, you may have to pass one off or just drop one.

> **"If you change the way you look at things, the things you look at change."**
>
> *Wayne Dyer*

36. Purchase a New Pair of Exercise Shoes

Sometimes the excitement of buying something new for a particular reason can stir up your motivation. If you purchase a pair of workout shoes specifically for exercising, they will serve as a constant reminder that you should be moving aerobically. Whenever you're looking for something in that closet, or moving something out of the way, those exercise shoes should make you feel a little more committed. Remember, you took the time to make the purchase, now take the time to put them to good use.

> **"I can feel the wind go by when I run. It feels good. It feels fast."**
>
> *Evelyn Ashford*

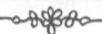

37. <u>Concentrate on One New Healthy Habit at a Time</u>

It's very easy to fall into the trap of trying to change multiple aspects of your life all at once in an attempt to lose weight faster. After all, it's not *that* difficult to eat more veggies and lean protein. Not *that* impossible to cut out the diet soda and drink more water or green tea. Not *that* overwhelming to lift weights several times a week, add some high intensity interval training, and get more sleep. That's because it *isn't* that difficult — provided you're already doing it.

When it comes to changing habits, most people use an all-or-nothing approach and become overwhelmed, which usually leads to failure. Getting fit — or learning any new skill — is a bit like juggling. If you begin by randomly throwing a dozen balls in the air, what's going to happen? Yes, they're all going to fall. But if you start with tossing one ball in the air, then eventually adding a second and then a third, you can master the skill. After figuring out what exercise schedule and eating plan is most feasible for your lifestyle, you can begin to phase in the additional steps to a healthier you, gradually and over time. Because it takes time and commitment to develop healthier habits, each month or two, focus on changing one habit at a time by either incorporating a healthy food into your diet or by adding a fitness challenge to help you become more active. The key is to not overwhelm yourself and feel the need to give it all up. Take one activity at a time and watch yourself accomplish all your goals in due time.

> *"Physcial fitness can neither be achieved by wishful thinking nor outright purchase."*
>
> *Joseph Pilates*

38. Improve Your Overall Health

Overall health is different from fitness health. Overall health is the search for enhanced quality of life, personal growth, and potential through positive lifestyle behaviors and attitudes. Guidelines for maintaining overall health require an accumulation of physical, emotional, intellectual, spiritual and interpersonal wellness. When enhancing your overall health:

- consider what's right with you.
- love yourself unconditionally.
- live in the present moment.
- exercise moderately by walking to work, dancing or raking leaves.
- don't take the challenges of life personally.
- eat a healthy diet.

- learn something new.
- grow intellectually.

> **"Doing something positive will help turn your mood around. When you smile, your body relaxes. When you experience human touch and interaction, it eases tension in your body."**
>
> *Simone Elkeles*

39. <u>Put Your Health Above Everyone Else</u>

First, take care of your health by doing things that are good for you and your mental stability. Women usually have problems putting themselves first because they perceive this as a selfish act. Putting your health above everyone else is not a selfish act. Rather it's an act of love. If you are unhealthy, you cannot effectively take care of your family or friends. Your body is a machine that works best when it is nourished with foods high in vitamins and minerals and it's stronger when it is strengthened with toning exercises and cardiovascular activities. When you put your health above everyone else, you are better able to take care of yourself and the ones you love.

> *"Women in particular need to keep an eye on their physical and mental health, because if we're scurrying to and from appointments and errands, we don't have a lot of time to take care of ourselves. We need to do a better job of putting ourselves higher on our own 'To-Do' list."*
>
> *Michelle Obama*

40. Don't Attempt to Eat Away Your Stress

It's easy to want to eat the first thing that's available when facing a stressful situation. We aim for comfort foods like macaroni & cheese, fried chicken, mashed potatoes, ice-cream and anything chocolate because they are tasty and pleasurable to eat. These foods have a mood-enhancing effect on our brains which makes us feel better when we're in a frazzled or stressed state. These same foods which may make us feel better in the short-term, also have a weight-enhancing affect on our bodies which usually makes us feel worse in the long-term. So, try hard to resist eating these foods when stressed because consequences like guilt, and depression usually follow the stress or binge-eating period.

When you're stressed, try distracting yourself by calling a friend, going to the movies, exercising or meditating. Soaking in a warm bath, getting a full-body massage or spending time with loved ones are a few other stress relievers that are good for the body and soul. However, if you have a strong desire to eat while you're in a stressful state, there are a host of great tasting, low-calorie, mood-lifting foods that can be eaten guilt-free. Snacks like: nut butter and fruit, greek yogurt and berries, fruit smoothies (with real fruit), protein bars, hummus, and plain home-popped popcorn are delicious alternatives and won't make you pack on the pounds. So, if you must eat when stressed, please consider the other low-fat alternatives, but more importantly, try very hard not to eat when stressed.

> *"To eat is a necessity, but to eat intelligently is an art."*
>
> *La Rochefoucauld*

41. Practice Patience

Losing weight never happens as quickly as you would like, but if you exercise and eat wisely, the pounds will begin to disappear, so just be patient. Patience is a person's ability to wait something out or endure something tedious, without getting riled up. When you begin your new lifestyle change, your body must first adjust by speeding up its metabolism and becoming stronger — so it's important to stay patient and focused! When you're patient and focused, you're able to push through sluggish and stressful times. Patience is knowing that you are doing something wonderful for your body, and your life, so HOLD ON and continue to push forward. Your patience will be rewarded.

> *"My advice is to go into something and stay with it until you like it. You can't like it until you obtain expertise in that work. And once you are an expert, it's a pleasure."*
>
> Milton Garland

42. Control Your Portion and Serving Sizes

The U.S. government developed *The Food Pyramid* as a guide for healthy eating, yet many people overestimate the serving sizes suggested by it. Even if you try hard to design your meals with a protein, vegetable and a starch, you may be surprised to learn that you've been supersizing those meals without even realizing it. With portion sizes so out of control these days, it may be hard to keep track of how much of which foods you should have each day, let alone how to measure it all. Now, you can easily visualize portion sizes, thanks to this "hand-y" guide from the United States Department of Agriculture.

1 cup = *A fist or cupped hand*
1 ounce of cheese = *A thumb*
1 - 2 ounces of snack food = *Handful*
3 ounces of meat = *Palm*
1 teaspoon = *Thumb Tip*
1 serving of fruit = *A tennis ball in the palm of your hand*

To see an actual serving size, measure your food for a typical meal according to these "hand-y" USDA guidelines, then put it on a plate. Now notice the difference between the suggested serving sizes and the heaping helpings to which we've become accustomed. For example, a serving size of chicken should be roughly the size and thickness of a deck of cards, not a whole skinless chicken breast. One serving of pasta is a half cup cooked — not one full bowl. And a serving of bread is one slice, not two (and preferably not white)! Your palm can be the perfect measuring tool since it is perfectly portioned just for you.

> *"Health is the thing that makes you feel that now is the best time of the year."*
>
> *Franklin P. Adams*

43. <u>Breathe Deeply</u>

Many people don't realize the powerful effects deep breathing has on their health and vitality. It is strange that something as fundamental as breathing goes unnoticed as being a powerful contributing factor to one's good health. Try this simple technique: Breathe in through your nose, hold the breath for a few seconds and then exhale through your mouth. When you breathe deeply, the air coming in through your nose fully fills your lungs, and you will notice that your lower belly rises. Spend five minutes, every one to two hours every day, inhaling and exhaling deeply with your hands on your ribs. You'll promote calmness and mental focus as well as renewed energy. As you exhale, try controlling your breathing by slowly counting from one to ten. Also try clearing your mind by mentally transporting yourself to a place that soothes your spirit. As basic as this may seem, these breathing exercises are effective ways of calming the mind and slowing down an elevated heart rate. These two things are essential for maintaining good overall health.

> **"If you don't design your own life plan, chances are you'll fall into someone else's plan. And guess what they have planned for you? Not much."**
>
> *Jim Rohn*

44. <u>Do it for You</u>

Don't exercise on impulse because you've seen beautiful pictures of a celebrity's fit body and want to emulate them. And definitely don't attempt to lose weight to get the attention of a woman or a man. It's okay to admire people who you view as beautiful, but the main person you want to be wonderful and look beautiful for is you. Certain images and expectations can be unrealistic and can start to diminish how you feel about yourself. Begin to take care of yourself because you really are worth it. Everything about you is magnificent and amazing, so exercise for you! Begin to appreciate your smile, age and curves — and whatever you decide to enhance or improve, remember to do it for you. When you lose weight and exercise for you, you are able to look yourself in the mirror and stand proud regardless of the outcome.

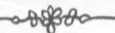

> **"Your goals minus your doubts, equals your reality."**
>
> *Ralph Marston*

45. Read Food Labels

All regulated processed foods include standardized nutrition information on their labels. These food labels show the serving sizes and the amount of fat, trans fat, cholesterol, sodium, total carbohydrate, dietary fiber, sugars and protein in every serving. By law, the words used on labels to describe foods mean the same thing for all foods. For example: <u>fat free</u> (must contain less than 0.5g of fat per serving) has the least amount of fat. <u>Low fat</u> and <u>very low fat</u> have a little more, and <u>reduced fat</u> or <u>less fat</u> always means that the food has 25% less fat than the regular version of the food. When it comes to sugar, try limiting added sugars to 24 grams a day (six teaspoons) if you eat 1,600 calories; 40 grams (10 teaspoons) for a 2,400-calorie diet; and 72 grams (18 teaspoons) for a 2,800-calorie diet. Remember to take a moment to read the nutrition label the next time you make a purchase.

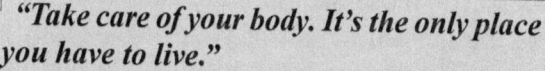

> *"Take care of your body. It's the only place you have to live."*
>
> *Jim Rohne*

46. Play to Your Preferences

Think of a non-fitness related activity you really love or loved years ago. Now, get creative and think of ways to combine that activity with a physical challenge. Finding the right activity can be as easy as getting in touch with the things you enjoyed doing when you were younger. Recapture a piece of your childhood, have a blast, and get in fabulous shape. For example, if you loved arts and crafts, take a nature walk and collect rocks, leaves and other objects for a collage to hang. Did you enjoy jumping rope or hula-hooping as a child? Health clubs and some workplace wellness centers provide jump-rope and hula-hoop classes. I've taught both, and my clients said that, "It brought back wonderful childhood memories." When your physical activity is combined with an activity you naturally adore, there is a good chance you'll do it more often. You can also try creating more active celebrations with your family. This can be as simple as having a picnic and playing outdoor sports, instead of having a sit down dinner. Remember, the best exercises aren't necessarily those that burn the most calories or take the most time out of your day — they're the activities you're most likely to do because you enjoy them. (Take the Physical Activity Enjoyment Scale Appendix D).

> *"The distance between who I am and who I want to be is separated only by my actions and words."*
>
> *Unknown-Internet*

47. Join a Health Club

How do you know if the health club you're about to join is the right one for you? Well, one of the first things you want to do is to take a tour before you join. How do you feel being there? Is it comfortable? Do you feel like you'll fit in with the crowd? Find out if you can get a trial membership before joining. Some gyms will offer at least a day, if not a week, to try it out before you join. While you're there, notice the people. How is the staff? Are they friendly and welcoming? Are they helpful? The more comfortable you are in the facility, the more likely you are to keep going back. Some health clubs are even offering clients "express" programs aimed at getting them in shape on a tight schedule. Some clubs offer 30-60 minute circuit and boot camp programs that allow clients to move swiftly from one fitness station to the next. Other clubs stay open 24 hours a day, seven days a week. In a health club you have the option to use the cardiovascular equipment (treadmills, bicycles, and elyptical machines) or you can participate in a group-led aerobic or circuit class, both of which offer high and low impact workouts (#26). Prefer no impact at all? Join a club with a pool and participate in a group aqua aerobics class. Group classes can be particularly helpful for people who don't have a lot of weight training or exercise experience. If you are uneasy about signing a contract, don't worry because many clubs have a pay-by-month membership plan. So, go ahead and visit a health club near you today; you'll be glad you did.

"The only bad workout is the one that didn't happen."

Unknown-Internet

48. Celebrate Your Success

If you're eating more fruits and vegetables this month than you were last month, celebrate your success. If you took the stairs rather than the elevator, celebrate your success. For your own personal growth, keep a daily and weekly success journal. Write down your "Success of the Day" for 30 days and you'll see amazing results. When you look for and celebrate your success, you'll notice more of it showing up in your life. You obviously can't change bad behaviors overnight, but you can celebrate every new behavior change that gets you closer to living a healthier lifestyle.

> *"The first and best victory is to conquer self."*
>
> *Plato*

49. Examine Your Risk Factors

While some risk factors for heart disease (such as heredity) can't be avoided, it's important to change those that can. Your overall wellness is largely determined by the decisions you make about how you live. Controlling your blood pressure, weight, stress level and smoking habits are critical to reducing your chances of developing heart disease. For example, if you know that diabetes is a family trait, then you know you need to eat a healthy diet and exercise often to reduce your risk of developing it. In addition to exercising, you should always get regular yearly check-ups that examine your overall health. Keep your doctor up to date on your fitness progress as well. He or she may have advice on ways to get and stay healthy inside and out. What you do today to strengthen your body can make the difference for a lifetime.

> *"Optimism is the faith that leads to achievement. Nothing can be done without hope and confidence."*
>
> *Helen Keller*

50. <u>Avoid Tobacco Products</u>

Smoking doesn't just affect the lungs. It affects your emotions and stress levels, your personal relationships, and all five of your senses. According to the University of Pittsburgh Cancer Institute, in as little as 48 hours of quitting, even your ability to smell and taste is enhanced. Within one year, heart attack risk is halved, and within 10 years, lung cancer risk is halved. The number one risk factor for cardiovascular disease that you can control is smoking. There's no doubt about it, kicking the smoking habit doesn't happen overnight. Research has found that most people try to quit five to seven times before they succeed. And unsuccessful "quit attempts," while frustrating, are actually part of the quitting process.

Many women avoid kicking the smoking habit because they fear putting on extra pounds. Believe me, the rewards of not smoking far outweigh the weight gain that can actually be controlled with a proper diet and exercise. Other benefits include the fact that your smoker's cough will begin to subside, and while you may have become accustomed to the smell, chances are the people around you haven't. In addition, you will have freed yourself from the mess, inconvenience, expense, and dependence of cigarette smoking. Avoiding tobacco products is a great start to the beginning of a healthier you.

> *"It is our attitude at the beginning of a difficult task which, more than anything else, will affect its successful outcome."*
>
> *William James*

51. Run for a Cause

Running is one of the most cost-effective forms of exercise there is. With no equipment to buy and no gym membership fees to pay, it's a great way to stay fit for little to no out-of-pocket expenses. If you're a beginner, you may want to check in with your doctor first. Next, you'll want to ease into a routine, so don't try to run three or four miles on your first day. Stretch, not just before or after, but also during a run. You can do this by including run-walk-stretch intervals. A wonderful motivator to run can be family, friends and co-workers. Organize a group to team up for the *Susan G. Komen Race for the Cure* or "The Color Run," a relatively new 5K race that focuses on healthiness and happiness more than timing and sponsors (www. thecolorrun.com). You can also join the Road Runners Club of America at www.rrca.org. It doesn't matter if it's a 5K, a 10K, or marathon, running for a cause can enhance your life and others.

> *"The doctor of the future will give no medication, but will interest his patients in the care of the human frame, in diet and in the cause and prevention of disease."*
>
> *Thomas A. Edison*

52. <u>Limit Your Sodium Intake</u>

It is possible to have delicious tasting meals without lots of salt by using a variety of herbs, spices and other seasonings. Basic natural seasonings like onion, garlic, lemon, vinegar, sugar, black pepper and parsley are readily found in most kitchens and can be used to improve the flavor of many different foods.

These flavorings enhance and add zest to the natural flavor of foods, making the missing salt less noticeable. Eating less sodium can also lower blood pressure, which may reduce the risk of heart disease. Sodium is something we need in our diets, but most of us use too much of it.

> *"Your past eating habits don't matter now. Focus on making better choices starting today."*
>
> *Unknown-Internet*

53. Ask for Gifts that Keep on Slimming

There are many smart fitness items that are perfect options for gifts — lightweight, easy to use, and can keep you in shape all year long. Of course, flowers and jewelry are always nice gifts during the holiday seasons, but why not include resistance bands on your holiday wish list? They are genius because they are lightweight, compact and versatile. You can also request a pocket pedometer, the device that digitally counts your steps. Studies show that pedometers inspire you to walk more. Another gift option is one of my new favorites: Reebok's Adjustable Dumbbells. It's taken a while for this new design to come with an affordable price tag, but it has finally happened. It won't clutter

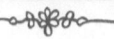

your living space and the cost is now under $100.00. You can also burn fat and strengthen your upper body with a crafty weight bearing jumprope. This convenient jumprope can be carried around in your briefcase, pocketbook or backpack. You can easily find any of these items online, or at an athletic store in your area.

> *"If you talked to your friends the way you talk to your body, you'd have no friends left."*
>
> *Marcia Hutchinson*

54. Add Muscle Toning to Your Workout Routine

Toning your muscles with weights or dumbbells not only creates the benefit of improved appearance, but skeletal health as well. That's why more and more women are turning to weightlifting as a relatively simple means of toning their bodies. Muscle toning is really the only type of exercise that targets specific body parts. The idea of muscle toning should not be mistaken for the bulky, muscle-bound Mr. or Mrs. Universe-style of body building. Instead, it's the kind of workout that, when done correctly a few times a week, gives the body a strong yet decidedly healthy look. If you're a beginner, a good way to gain muscle is to

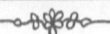

start with 30 minutes of toning, with 5-10 pound barbells, three times per week. Once the 5-10 pound weights begin to feel less challenging, challenge yourself by increasing your weights by two to five pounds gradually.

> *"Always do your best. What you plant now, you will harvest later."*
>
> *Maria Robinson*

55. <u>Be Aggressive</u>

If you want to achieve anything in life, you must become aggressive. You cannot achieve much by being passive. Passivity derives from fear. For many, fear can be an obstacle, but for you, let it be an illusion. You may think something is standing in your way, but trust me, nothing is really there. Don't be afraid to change your lifestyle just because you have to step out of your comfort zone. Be aggressive and pursue a healthy lifestyle as though your life depends on it – because it does!

> *"Even if you fall on your face, you're still moving forward."*
>
> *Victor Kiam*

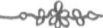

56. <u>Enhance Your Spiritual Wellness</u>

Spiritual wellness means different things to different people, but generally it is associated with enhancing your coping skills. It involves developing a set of guiding beliefs, principles and values that give purpose and meaning to your life to help you cope with tough times. Spiritual wellness can bond people together through compassion, love, forgiveness, and self-sacrifice. It can make you more aware of your personal values or it can help you clarify what they are. Living according to values means making the best choice for you morally, spiritually and emotionally and acting on it, rather than doing nothing. You are already on a journey of self-fulfillment and overall enhancement, so take a little time to heighten your spiritual wellness, too. You'll be glad you did.

> *"We are not human beings learning to be spiritual, we are spiritual beings learning to be human."*
>
> *Jacqueline Small*

57. <u>Don't Make Excuses</u>

One of the most important steps to losing weight is to stop making excuses about why you cannot. Part of being committed to a healthier lifestyle is taking responsibility for your actions instead of making excuses for them. Whenever you are trying to achieve anything, there will be roadblocks, but obstacles don't have to deter you. Figure out how to go through them, or work around them and move forward. When you truly value your health, you will devote time to exercise and eating healthier. Don't make excuses for why you can't; give reasons for why you can.

"It's not supposed to be easy. Disciplined people succeed; undisciplined people don't...Nothing changes by doing what's fun and easy."

Tom Venuto

58. <u>Read More Health-Related Topics</u>

Reading is educational, entertaining and downright exciting. Take responsibility for your health by developing the habit of reading and learning more about the importance of diet and exercise. Learn more about the magnificent body in all its shapes, colors and sizes by reading topics related to health and wellness. The more you know, the more inclined you are to take better care of yourself. It may take some discipline at first, but it will offer magnificent benefits in the long run as you become healthier, more aware, and ageless.

> *"Be kinder than necessary, for everyone you meet is fighting some kind of battle. Live simply, love generously, care deeply, speak kindly…and the rest will fall in place."*
>
> Charles Swindall

59. Practice Affirmations

One way of cultivating the positive is to systematically repeat positive thoughts, or affirmations, to yourself. For example, if you have low self-esteem, you might repeat sentences like, "I approve of and accept myself completely." If you find yourself criticizing your appearance, you might repeat, "I am perfect, strong and beautiful."

The affirmation process is an interesting one because when you're trying to change a thought or feeling, it may take you repeating a statement 5, 10 or 20 times before you actually believe it. I practice affirmations often and I remember one time in particular repeating a statement quickly and with purpose at least 15-20 times until the negative thought or feeling diminished. Saying affirmations to yourself every day can make them automatic as they can help you change the way you see yourself. But remember, it's not just about saying these affirmations — it's about believing them. Don't just say that you are beautiful. Believe that you are beautiful. Don't just say that you are smart. Believe that you are smart. Don't just say you are unstoppable. Believe...and then BE UNSTOPPABLE! Practice affirmations and know that you can and will accomplish your goals, dreams and objectives.

> *"You must do the thing you think you cannot do."*
>
> *Eleanor Roosevelt*

60. Shut Down Your Kitchen

Do you shut down your kitchen at night? If not, late night snacking could be keeping you from getting the results you want. Food is fuel, and food eaten right before bedtime when your energy is at its lowest becomes stored fat. Try eating your large meals, or preferably mini-meals during the day when your body is able to burn more energy. During early evening hours your meals should be lighter and healthier than during the day. Once you've eaten your last meal, preferably 3-4 hours before bed, shut down your kitchen and brush your teeth. Brushing your teeth tells your brain that not only has the kitchen shut down for the evening, but the overall consumption of food has as well; because you definitely don't want to ruin that clean mouth and fresh breath for a midnight snack.

"Remember: Fat lasts longer than flavor."

Unknown-Internet

---

61. Go Easy on the Gravy, Dips and Sauces

One tablespoon of gravy made from turkey drippings can contain up to 70 calories, and one ladle as much as 800. The same applies to high calorie dips, salad dressings and cheesy sauces. If you use the gravy packet in the supermarket aisle, you're okay, because you only add water and the average packet is only 20 calories. A prepared gravy in a can or jar, however, is higher in fat and calorie content. If you use

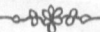

drippings from your meat to prepare your gravy the homemade way, be sure to scoop the fat from the top. Use dips and sauces sparingly or substitute them with lower-calorie items like yogurt, cottage cheese dips, lemon juice, tomato salsa or vinaigrette dressings.

> *"A man too busy to take care of his health is like a mechanic too busy to take care of his tool."*
>
> Spanish proverb

62. Cook the Low-Fat Way

You can cook the low-fat way by baking, braising, broiling, steaming or grilling. This healthy way of cooking will change the way you and your family approach food for a lifetime. Use nonstick cooking spray instead of butter or oil; or at least choose liquid oils over solid fats (preferably canola or olive oil). Choose lean meats and skinless poultry over pork and watch your serving sizes carefully. Coat chicken and fish in breadcrumbs, rather than batter, and bake them instead of frying them. Substitute two meat dishes each week with fish or vegetarian meals. You can also stir-fry with veggies, using only a teaspoon of oil per person. Oven-fry potatoes instead of making or buying french fries, and use half the amount of oil called for in recipes for main dishes like biscuits, cornbread and muffins. These simple steps can improve your day when you decide to cook the low-fat way.

> *"Enjoy losing weight. Enjoy eating healthy, delicious food. Do not wait until you reach your destination to feel good. Take as much happiness and joy as you can from your weight loss journey."*
>
> *Harry Papas*

63. Weight Loss Stalls? Don't Panic!

Okay, so now you're doing everything right. You are cutting back on your food consumption, you've increased your physical activity, and yet, the scale hasn't budged much. It's important to understand that when switching to a healthier lifestyle, your weight loss may inexplicably stop, no matter how hard you try to drop another pound. Don't panic and don't get discouraged. This is totally normal. You may still be losing weight, but your body is readjusting its level of fat to lean muscle. Just stay focused, and DON'T PANIC!

> *"Nobody can go back and start a new beginning, but anyone can start today and make a new ending."*
>
> *Maria Robinson*

64. Your Eyes are Bigger than Your Stomach

Your eyes are actually bigger than your stomach, so eat until you're satisfied — not stuffed — and save the rest for later. It doesn't take nearly as much food as you think to curb your appetite and meet your body's need for fuel. All the extra helpings you eat after you're full get stored as reserve energy — otherwise known as fat. If you have a problem knowing when to say no, try biting into a pickle or lemon. Neither has any calories, and the sour taste will help to curb your appetite. Don't have either? Brush your teeth before a meal, this too will help to curb your appetite and assist your eyes with appearing a little smaller than your stomach.

> *"Tell me what you eat and I will tell you what you are."*
>
> *Jean Anthelme Brillat-Savarin*

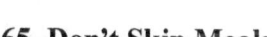

65. <u>Don't Skip Meals</u>

If you're skipping meals to lose weight, you're doing yourself a disservice. When you skip meals, your body senses a food shortage and slows down your metabolism to conserve energy. The absence of food causes the stomach to secrete a hormone called ghrelin. Ghrelin is referred to as "the hunger hormone." It's an enzyme produced by the stomach lining cells that stimulates appetite. It exerts its effects by slowing down fat utilization and increasing appetite. Without consistent food consumption, ghrelin levels remain elevated for extended periods of time, increasing the desire to eat. As a result, your body *stores* calories instead of *burning* them, hindering any weight loss. When you finally eat, you will tend to over-eat, which is what leads to weight gain. Frequent meals counteract these negative effects (#15). Blood sugar is better regulated and because there is an almost constant flow of food into the stomach, the hunger-inducing effects of ghrelin are suppressed, reducing the urge to binge-out.

> *"Our health always seems much more valuable after we lose it."*
>
> *Unknown-Internet*

66. <u>Purchase Exercise Equipment</u>

Having a piece of exercise equipment in your home allows you the freedom to exercise at your leisure. It also gives you the freedom to multi-task. For a person who works at the office from 8a.m. until 6p.m., having home exercise equipment may be the only way to structure the environment so that regular physical activity is an option. Of course, simply having exercise equipment in the environment does not necessarily provide the motivation for the individual to actually use it. For that, it may be important for the individual to learn to pair leisure activities he/she likes and perceives as important (such as watching the evening news, reading the newspaper, or listening to music) with use of the home exercise equipment. Before purchasing a piece of equipment, take a test drive. You can do this at a local gym, recreation center, retailer or even at a friend's place. You may also want to check out consumer and fitness magazines that rate exercise equipment. This will give you an idea of how well the product performs before you spend your money. And, last but not least, know what your goals are. Are you trying to build strength, increase flexibility, improve endurance or just become healthier? Use these guidelines to help you decide which piece of exercise equipment is right for you and will provide you with your desired results.

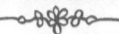

> *"If you wait for perfect conditions, you'll never get anything done."*
>
> The Bible, Ecclesiastes 11:4 (NLT)

67. <u>Purchase or Borrow Exercise DVDs</u>

Exercise DVDs are some of the most popular weight loss instruments around these days. They can recreate the energy of a health club aerobics class, and their strategies are good for improving your heart, flexibility and strength. In fact, you can go to any Walmart, Target or Kmart store and find a section of various workout DVDs. One of the main benefits of exercise DVDs is that they allow you to work out in the comfort of your own home. Working out at a gym is a great way to get in shape, but exercising alongside a number of people is not for everyone. If you are feeling self-conscious about your body, then you would probably prefer to exercise in private. Workout DVDs also give you the opportunity to set your workout time at hours that are convenient for you. This can be a particularly important benefit if you have a hectic lifestyle and you have a hard time finding exercise classes that fit into your schedule. Before your purchase, borrow one from your local library at no cost. You can even download one straight to your cable box. First, choose a

DVD that matches your current fitness level. This will help so you don't get discouraged by exercises that are too difficult or too easy. If you like grooving to the beat, then choose a Zumba DVD. If you prefer aggressive workouts, then there are boot-camp and kickboxing DVDs available as well. Exercise DVDs are fun, can prevent boredom, are convenient, and can add variety to your workout.

> *"It's never a question of can you, but will you?"*
>
> *Unknown-Internet*

68. Exercise with Household Items

Do not let NOT having weights or equipment deter you from exercising at home. Your couch and coffee tables are perfect props for working out — anything from single-leg squats to push-ups. Look at elastic household items, such as a bunji cord as essential strength training equipment. Stretchy cords are excellent options for bicep curls and can help encourage good form, especially if you're new to exercising. You can either make handles for the ends of the cord or just tie a knot, leaving space to loop your hands through.

To create an inexpensive set of weights, fill your empty milk cartons and water bottles with sand, rocks or liquid (be sure to secure the tops with tape) or use your groceries just as they are. One full gallon-sized jug of milk weighs about 8.5 pounds, which is perfect for giving your arms a good workout. Laundry detergent bottles are also good dumbbell alternatives. A 72-ounce bottle of detergent weighs about 5 pounds. Canned goods come in a variety of sizes and are also easy to hold as weights. You can tighten your butt and thighs by holding your weights by your sides and completing as many walking lunges as you can (the length of my home allows me to complete 20 in one direction).

Complete basic exercises like bicep curls for front arm strength. Place your hands, palms facing upwards in front of your thighs and bend your elbows to curl the canned goods to shoulder level. Slowly lower, and repeat. For the back of the arms, complete at least ten tricep kick-backs. Have your palms facing your buttocks, elbows bent and by your side close to your waist. Keep your upper arms still, extend your lower arms down towards the buttocks to lower the cans and repeat.

Strengthen your abdominal muscles by placing your feet beneath the sofa and complete as many sit-ups as you can. If you're stretching or exercising on the floor, use a towel or blanket if you don't have a mat. And why not use the original stair climber – the stairs! Running up and down the stairs is a great workout. Exercising with household items doesn't have to be a chore, instead it can be fun, low-cost and effective.

> *"I am in the pursuit of awesomeness, excellence is the bare minimum."*
>
> *Kanye West*

69. Get a Good Night's Sleep

Are you getting enough sleep? Half of all adults are not, yet adequate rest is as vital to health and peak performance as exercise and good nutrition. The first step to improving the quality of your rest is finding out how much sleep you need. How much sleep is enough for you? While sleep requirements vary slightly from person to person, most healthy adults need at least eight hours of sleep each night to function at their best.

A study from Oregon State University found that at least 150 minutes of moderate to vigorous exercise per week improved sleep quality by 65 percent. Other research has shown that your mother was right — you should tidy up your sheets: people who made their bed every day were 19 percent more likely to report a better night's rest. I picked this habit up a few years ago and I'm still amazed at how much better I feel and sleep when I see a well-made bed. If you keep a regular sleep schedule, by going to bed and getting up at the same time each day, you will feel much more refreshed and energized than if you sleep even the same number of hours but at different times. This holds true even if you alter your sleep schedule by only an hour or two. Consistency is vitally important.

Another way to get a good night's sleep is to add one cup of whole wheat pasta to your dinner a few nights a week. It contains 38% of your daily value of magnesium. Magnesium has a relaxing effect on the muscles and the nervous system. If you need an alarm clock to wake up on time, you may need to set an earlier bedtime, because if you're getting enough sleep you should wake up naturally without an alarm. And last but definitely not least, watch television on the sofa instead of the bed. Every minute you spend awake and out of bed increases your need for deep sleep. If you find yourself getting sleepy way before your bedtime, get off the couch and do something mildly stimulating to avoid falling asleep too early, such as washing the dishes, calling a friend, or getting clothes ready for the next day. Sleeping better and longer will help you wake up with a pep in your step and a desire to conquer all of your dreams and goals.

> *"The higher your energy level, the more efficient your body. The more efficient your body, the better you feel and the more you will use your talent to produce outstanding results."*
>
> Anthony Robbins

70. <u>Make Fitness a Habit</u>

Let's face it: it's not all that difficult to start a fitness routine. After all, most of us have tried it more than once. The trouble, of course, comes with sticking with it. All too often, our initial enthusiasm and energy wanes, we get distracted by other things going on in our lives, or we don't think we're seeing results quickly enough — so we throw in the towel. The chronic physiological improvements associated with cardiovascular training usually take 8-12 weeks. Detraining effects start to occur in as few as 12 to 21 days. This means that you begin to lose what you've worked so hard to achieve in a very short period of time; which is why it's very important to make fitness a habit. Two important keys to making fitness a habit are: 1.) Do something you enjoy, and 2.) Include it into your daily routine. Long-term exercisers (who had been working out for an average of 13 years) were asked by researcher David Klein, PhD to rank what motivated them to keep up with their regimes. Their answers might surprise you. The exercisers were not as concerned with large muscles and tight abs as they were with feeling good and being healthy. Cardiovascular fitness gains are generally lost faster than muscular fitness gains, but muscles can atrophy, losing tone and strength if you don't continue training them. So make fitness a habit and watch your overall health, level of fitness and confidence rise.

"The chains of habit are generally too small to be felt until they are too strong to be broken."

Samuel Johnson

71. <u>Take the Stairs</u>

Climbing the stairs used to be an option only if the elevator was not working. Today, more and more people are recognizing the importance of taking the stairs. When you take the stairs instead of the elevator, you're including fitness into your daily schedule and strengthening your heart and overall endurance without doing anything to change your routine. This form of exercise is good for your heart as it can lower your bad cholesterol levels and raise your good cholesterol levels. It relieves tension and stress and can lower the risk of hypertension and

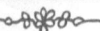

diseases that are related to heart health. It's also a great way to accomplish a few things at once. You are already at work or taking care of business, you don't need a sitter, and you're getting fit. It's sometimes even much faster to take the stairs, especially during peak times when elevators take a long time to arrive on the floor of your location. So, fight the temptation of walking through those elevator doors and walk to the staircase instead. Your heart will be glad you did.

> *"It's actually pretty simple. Either you do it, or you don't."*
>
> *Unknown-Internet*

72. <u>Avoid Supermarket Temptations</u>

Ever been to the supermarket to buy a carton of milk, only to head to the checkout line with a handful of items? You can't avoid the grocery store altogether; you have to get food, after all. However, you can learn to shop smarter and avoid some of the enticing products that can ruin your diet.

Some of the best ways to avoid supermarket temptations include making a list and sticking to it, taking market trips *after* you've eaten (so you're not tempted to purchase out of hunger), and lastly, sticking to your budget. Also, once you've made the list of the things you need to purchase, take the estimated amount of cash. Paying by card means there's no limit, allowing you to add unnecessary items to your original list. By leaving the card at home, you are minimizing the opportunity for impulsive purchases. Retailers actually arrange their stores to encourage impulse (and often unhealthy) buys. Just think about the candy bars right by the cash register, or the aroma of fresh baked goods that greet you as soon as you enter the door. Also, avoid "free samples." This little taste often winds up triggering an unnecessary purchase.

> *"Willpower is a muscle. The more you use it, the stronger it gets."*
>
> *Unknown-Internet*

73. Beware of Diet and Exercise Saboteurs

Diet and exercise saboteurs wear many masks. Unfortunately, they can be a spouse, parent, co-worker or friend who secretly or subconsciously sabotages your efforts to lose weight and get fit. Some view your success as a mirror of their own failures. Others fear that you'll change emotionally as you become more self assured and physically confident. If you learn to recognize diet and exercise saboteurs while they're in action, you'll be less likely to let them derail you from your goals.

Office jobs tend to celebrate special events with cookies, cakes or doughnuts, but instead of giving in to the temptations, tell co-workers you're trying to change and ask if they want to join you. If that doesn't work, avoid the break room altogether and bring your own meals and snacks. If your significant other asks you to go out to dinner before your work out, politely agree to spend time with them after your workout and not before. And if someone makes a negative or discouraging remark on how, "You're conceited now that you've lost weight," or that, "You need to stop exercising because you're getting so thin," don't take it personally and don't let him or her get you down. Remember, the changes you're making will not make everyone happy, but give yourself permission to make them anyway.

> *"The difference between a successful person and others is not a lack of strength, not a lack of knowledge, but rather a lack in will."*
>
> *Vince Lombardi*

74. <u>Always Have a "Plan B"</u>

Learning how to become flexible when life throws you a curve ball is extremely important and probably one of the most important tools you can take into an exercise program. Momentum can be a powerful thing – whether it's working with you or against you. When you have a specific plan to follow for your diet and exercise, you have to anticipate days of bad weather, afternoons when the gym is overcrowded, and nights out with your friends where the meal choices are less than optimal.

Setbacks are inevitable, as they are a part of life, so it's important to always have a Plan B. Sometimes what throws you off track is your own doing (you overslept, over-indulged on vacation, or smoked the cigarette that triggered the relapse). Other times it's out of your control (you accidentally injured yourself or a family member is ill). Once that one day is missed, it makes skipping the second day much easier, and before you know it, a whole month has gone by and you "just can't get back into it." The healthier you are, the better able you are to withstand the trials and tribulations of life. If you enjoy jogging outside during the warm months, be sure to have access to a gym or fitness facility to use their treadmills during the cooler months. If your Zumba class is cancelled, have the address of another class location on hand, or maybe have a Zumba DVD at home to work out to. If walking through your neighborhood becomes a bit boring, don't stop walking. Instead, go to your neighborhood park or bike trail. You may even want to drive to a popular walking trail and meet other walkers. Having a Plan B removes the excuses and keeps you on track.

> *"The difference between someone who is in shape and someone who is not in shape, is the individual who is in shape works out even when they do not want to."*
>
> *Unknown-Internet*

75. Eat Fruits and Vegetables Every Day

A recent study found that 75% of U.S. residents don't eat the recommended three cups of vegetables and two cups of fruits daily. Fresh fruits and vegetables are the cornerstone of a healthy diet which helps to reduce the effects of aging. It's been proven over time that the vitamins, minerals and antioxidants in fruits and vegetables can help reduce the risk of cancer, heart disease, high blood pressure and type II diabetes. Over the past 30 years or so, researchers have developed a solid base of science to back up what mothers have preached for generations: *You must eat your fruits and vegetables.* The latest research suggests that the biggest payoff from eating fruits and vegetables goes to your heart. In fact, the ubiquitous 5 A Day slogan which encouraged the consumption of at least five portions of fruits and vegetables each day, has been changed to Fruits & Veggies — More Matters. This statement was supported in part by the National Cancer Institute and is now seen in produce aisles and magazine ads all over the country. Here's a tip: set time aside to wash, chop and divide your vegetables and fruits into snack size servings that will allow you to grab and go. People whose diets are rich in fresh fruits and vegetables have more energy and are less likely to gain weight. The latest Dietary Guidelines for Americans attempted to simplify the government advice in this way: At least half of your plate should be filled with fruits and/or veggies.

> *"Let your food be your medicine, and your medicine be your food."*
>
> Hippocrates

76. Become Your Own Cheerleader

The energy and enthusiasm of a cheerleader is necessary when handling the radical emotional changes required to raise self-esteem and move to higher levels. Use this analogy to handle adversity: If you don't feel motivated or enthusiastic, then pretend! The strange thing is that within a few minutes, you might actually start to feel motivated or enthusiastic for real. It is very easy to say, "I can't do something." This negative thinking or response takes no energy or drive and it will also get you nowhere. Try telling yourself you CAN do something. And say it with enthusiasm. Positive reinforcement will get you where you want to go. Force the clutter and negative thoughts out of your head and fill it with new inspirations that will put "pep in your step" and a positive attitude in your spirit. Being your own cheerleader isn't silly; it's smart and contagious.

> *"Do you think, 'I can't. I don't want to. I'm feeling stressed,' or 'I can! I want to! I'm feeling exhilarated!'?"*
>
> *Unknown Internet*

77. <u>You Can Survive the Snack Attack</u>

It's 10p.m., it's bed time, and you are craving a snack. But what do you eat? Or *should* you eat? You may be surprised to know that it's actually not the snacking alone that is the problem; it's what you're snacking on that matters most. Snacks can be a terrific way to satisfy your hunger and speed up your metabolism, but it's important to pay attention to what you eat. Stay away from foods that are high in calories and saturated fats. Think healthy — a piece of fruit, or fresh vegetables with fat-free dip are low-calorie snacks that can still hit the spot. To ensure healthy snacking while at work or on the go, prepare your snacks in advance. Keep your snacks with you, give yourself a variety of choices, and remember to read food labels (#45).

To survive the Snack Attack, you certainly do not want to keep snacks in your bedroom, and you want to try very, very hard to keep high fat snacks out of your home altogether. If you practice the mini-meal concept (#15), you can regulate your blood sugars and keep from overeating throughout the day. This way, that urge to have a snack can fit nicely into a healthy eating routine. Also remember to stock your refrigerator with a variety of fruits, and vegetables, and your cabinets with whole grain cereals and snack mixes made from popcorn, oats and whole wheat. Surviving the Snack Attack can make snacking great for the entire family when good snack food choices are made.

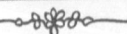

"Whether you think you can or you think you can't, you're right."

Henry Ford

78. <u>Your Body Needs Rest to Perform Its Best</u>

While regular exercise is important if you want to see physical progress, you shouldn't feel that you can't take a day or two off when starting a new exercise regime. Your body needs time to adapt to the physiological changes that will occur; this is why allowing time to recover from workouts is so important. Remember, the "building-up part" (muscle repair and rebuild) happens after the exercise is over, not during the workouts. Resting also aids in the removal of metabolic waste products such as lactic acid (the chemical responsible for muscle soreness and fatigue). In other words, what you do *outside* the gym for your recovery is just as important as what you do *in* the gym, when it comes to changing your body. Think of rest to perform your best!

"Your fitness is 100% mental! Your body won't go where your mind doesn't push it!"

Unknown-Internet

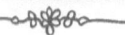

79. Perform Calf Raises While Working

The gastrocnemius (calf muscle) gives shape to a woman's legs, so why not exercise them regularly as you complete your daily chores and duties. Calf raises can be performed while sitting or while standing, while brushing your teeth, combing your hair, sitting at your desk or just performing routine activities around your home. To perform an ideal calf raise, wear tennis shoes, flat soft-soled shoes, or no shoes at all. When performing a calf raise while standing, lift up onto the balls of your feet with your knees slightly bent, lower your heels back onto the floor and repeat throughout the day as often as possible. If you are sitting, raise your feet up as high as you can until you are on the balls of both feet, hold for 3 seconds and plant your heel back onto the floor. Repeat at least 10 times.

"Look to your health; and if you have it, praise God and value it next to conscience; for health is the second blessing that we mortals are capable of, a blessing money can't buy."

Izaak Walton

80. <u>Avoid the Scale</u>

Step away from the scale! Focusing on weight loss by the numbers alone can derail your efforts. Weight naturally fluctuates, even when you're doing everything right, and the reasons may vary completely. They can be anything from your food ingestion the night before, the time of day, your day's activities, or your body's water level. While the scale is good for giving a general idea of your weight, you should avoid the scale because it can also be the most discouraging and frustrating part of your weight-loss plan. Besides, you don't need a scale to tell you what type of shape you're in because there is a good chance you already know. Stay off the scale and determine how good you look by how good you feel, not by numbers. When you first begin a fitness regime, you lose inches before total body weight, so getting on a scale too often or too soon can give you a false reality. Instead, acknowledge small milestones along the way — like looser jeans or shaving a minute or two off your walking pace. The reality is that your body is changing daily so enjoy the process and avoid the scale.

"Change your thoughts and you will change your world."

Norman Vincent Peale

81. <u>Get a Physical Examination</u>

Getting a full physical examination is a great first step to being aware of your physical health and taking action. A physical examination, also known simply as a "physical," is a process by which a physician examines various organ systems and other parts of your body. It is a standard tool to diagnose disease and monitor overall health. Getting a physical examination can help prevent diseases before they occur or deal with them before they become dangerous. This way, you know where you stand before starting an exercise program. Your physician may also be able to advise you on the areas that you should concentrate on more in your exercise program, or alert you to the areas you should avoid overexerting. For example, if your physician diagnoses you with asthma but you still want to exercise and work out consistently, they will know what type of medication to provide you with and may be able to offer advice on when and how to exercise to avoid an asthma attack. Talk to your doctors — they are your friends.

"Our health always seems much more valuable after we lose it."

Unknown-Internet

82. <u>Dance Like Nobody's Watching</u>

Have a fun and fabulous time at home dancing like nobody's watching. Have fun with it, pretend to be whomever you like, and burn calories at the same time. Imagine you're on "Fame" like Debbie Allen, or salsa like Jennifer Lopez. No partner is needed and your focus is fun, fun, fun as you burn calories, calories, calories. This is something positive for your mind, body and soul. Be inspired to move by rejuvenating daily with a dose of dance. Start your morning with your favorite music and your very own dance party. Be free, look good, feel great, and dance like nobody's watching.

> *"Today, I will be happier than a bird with a french fry."*
>
> *Toni Nelson*

83. <u>Get Healthier Skin</u>

Three important lifestyle habits necessary for clear skin are consistent and adequate sleep, good hydration, and regular exercise. Getting good rest will always leave the body and face refreshed and healthy. One only has to look in the mirror after a night of restless sleep to see bags under the eyes, dark circles, and acne. And no one wants that. Hydration is also very important, as it removes waste from the body and helps keep your system and skin clean. So, drink eight or more eight-ounce glasses of water per day to keep your skin healthy. Last, but certainly not least, is regular exercise. It's important to include cardiovascular activities into your schedule as it helps the body maintain good blood flow and cardiovascular health. All three of these habits done simultaneously will result in your body becoming increasingly efficient with toxin removal which will reflect radiant skin. Remember, it's easier to have healthier skin if you think of it as a lifestyle and not something that comes in a bottle.

"We must become the change we want to see."

Gandhi

84. Lower Your Blood Pressure

Since high blood pressure has no symptoms, almost half of the estimated 50 million Americans with hypertension don't know their blood pressure is high according to the American Heart Association. When your pressure is checked, you will receive two numbers. The first (top) number is the systolic pressure. It is the pressure in your arteries when your heart squeezes. The second (bottom) number is the diastolic pressure. It is the pressure in your arteries when your heart relaxes. High blood pressure is defined as a consistent reading of 140/90 or greater. Although the specific causes of high blood pressure often can't be determined, doctors have identified several risk factors that increase the likelihood of developing hypertension:

- Age - High blood pressure is more likely to develop after age 35.
- Obesity- Individuals weighing 30% or more above their ideal body weight are at increased risk of hypertension.
- Lack of Exercise - An inactive lifestyle can contribute to obesity and hypertension.
- Race - African Americans tend to be at a higher risk than other ethnicities including Caucasians and Hispanic Americans.
- Heredity - Hypertension can run in families.
- Diet - Diets containing high amounts of salt and fat can cause increased blood pressure in some individuals.
- Alcohol - Regular, heavy alcohol use can be related to high blood pressure.
- Diabetes - Diabetes that is not well controlled by medications places individuals at increased risk.

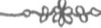

"Occassionally, in life, there are those moments of unutterable fulfillment which cannot be completely explained by those symbols called words. Their meanings can only be articulated by the inaudible language of the heart."

Martin Luther King, Jr.

85. Prepare Healthy Meals with Your Family

Beyond the benefit of good health and nutrition, family meals provide a valuable opportunity to reconnect on an emotional level with the people you love. When I was a child, family meals were so important that if you didn't eat with the family, you didn't eat at all. My siblings and I were not only a part of the food preparation process, but we also had specific duties. I scaled fish and cleaned a variety of fresh greens, all while in middle school. Getting your teenager involved may be a little more difficult but the benefits can far outway the difficulty. Cooking with your child can improve parent-child relationships, decrease power struggles, and boost healthy eating habits. If you have younger children, you can get them involved by helping to set the table or by measuring dry ingredients. Children will get a sense of pride from helping to prepare the meal, and will also be more inclined to eat it. Research shows that children who eat family meals consume more fruits and vegetables, eat less saturated fat, and have an overall higher-quality diet. My siblings and I are definitely representatives of this research. You, too, can enjoy quick and healthy meals with your family, and they, too, can have memories to cherish for a lifetime.

> *"The food you eat can be either the safest and most powerful form of medicine or the slowest form of poison."*
>
> *Ann Wigmore*

86. Know Your Fitness Personality

Get motivated and beat exercise burnout by matching your fitness personality. Your fitness personality is what gets you up and moving. What time of day do you feel most comfortable dancing, running or stretching? You don't need to spend multiple hours at a gym to accomplish any of these activities, but you must determine what time of day works best for you. For instance, if working out helps you to unwind after a long day, you may want to make arrangements to keep the children at the sitter's an hour longer and head straight to the gym. If your fitness personality is geared toward morning workouts, you will never be satisfied exercising after work, so wake up an hour earlier. If you're a mid-day energizer bunny, focus on exercising during your lunch break. If you worry about sweating during your afternoon workout sessions, try exercises that don't usually allow heavy panting like yoga, pilates, toning, or stretching. Once you determine your exercise personality you can actually create a workout routine that fits into your schedule rather than against it.

> *"I don't work hard because I hate my body, I work out because I love it."*
>
> *Unknown-Internet*

87. <u>Beware of Impulsive Vending Machine Snacking</u>

On March 23, 2010, President Barack Obama signed the health care reform legislation into law. Section 4205 of the Patient Protection and Affordable Care Act of 2010 requires vending machine operators who own or operate 20 or more vending machines to disclose calorie content for certain items. This is good news if you often find yourself visiting your conveniently located vending machine at work. While you should still limit your visits to the vending machine, if you can't fight the temptation, be sure to choose

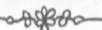

an item that is listed as a low-calorie snack. You may also want to keep a personal stash of fresh or dried fruits and vegetables at your desk — this will help to keep those vending machine visits to a minimum (#75 & #77). Working eight hours a day without snacking is almost impossible for anyone, including me, but if you make wise selections, these vending machine visits won't appear to be as dreadful or unhealthy. If you are unaware of how often you are snacking, try keeping a food and snack diary. This will help put your snacking into perspective and help you to stay clear of impulsive vending machine visits.

> *"Most of us think we don't have enough time to exercise. What a distorted paradigm! We don't have time not to. We're talking about three to six hours a week — or a minimum of thirty minutes a day, every other day. That hardly seems an inordinate amount of time considering the tremendous benefits in terms of the impact on the other 162-165 hours of the week."*
>
> Stephen Covey

88. <u>Become a Picky Eater</u>

Many of us have a friend or two who requests salads and fruit cups when everyone else orders burgers and french fries. When this happens, the person is seen as dieting or depriving themselves of a wonderful meal. So what do we do? We start calling these people health nuts or picky eaters. However, you, too, should become a picky eater. Make a rule to eat veggies at every meal and snack, not just at lunch and dinner. Throw some spinach, broccoli, or beans into your smoothie or snack on celery or carrot sticks smeared with nut butter. For lunch, go for an enormous salad (light on the dressing), and for dinner have at least three different kinds of veggies, such as asparagus, yellow peppers, and broccoli. Increasing the variety of natural foods in your diet not only keeps you fired up about eating healthy foods, it also means your body is getting a greater variety of vitamins and other important nutrients. This eating plan will help fight off killer diseases such as heart disease, stroke, cancer, and diabetes.

Becoming a picky eater isn't boring or dull, instead, it's invigorating, wholesome and can keep you "fit as a fiddle." Eating this way may now earn you the reputation of a picky or conscious eater, but it will also reduce your risk of becoming obese which is emerging as the second leading cause of preventable death in the U.S. Which would you rather be?

> **"You can set yourself up to be sick, or you can choose to stay well."**
>
> *Wayne Dyer*

89. Be Vain

Go on, check yourself out in that plate glass window, your full length mirror, or on the back of that dinner knife. Reflecting on your reflection can count as good preventive medicine. When you pay close attention to the subtle changes in your appearance, you're more likely to spot changes and early signs that can be of importance. Touch yourself all over before and during your shower — does everything feel normal? Sometimes your complexion can serve as a reminder of whether or not you need more water in your diet, or maybe you notice that your hips are getting wider. STOP. Schedule a physical examination right away, and check out your diet and exercise schedule to see where you've been slacking and do something about it. The sooner you pick up on the clues, the faster you can take the right steps to getting and staying healthier. Being vain is good for your self esteem and your overall health as well.

"Noble and great. Courageous and determined. Faithful and fearless. That is who you are and who you have always been. And understanding it can change your life, because this knowledge carries a confidence that cannot be duplicated any other way."

Sheri L. Dew

90. <u>Smell Before You Eat and Eat Slowly</u>

Research from the Smell and Taste Treatment and Research Foundation in Chicago, IL suggests that the aroma of certain foods can trick your brain into thinking your stomach is already full. Two examples: peppermint and banana. Believe it — your appetite is controlled by the brain. You can keep a raging appetite under control by slicing up a green apple and simply smelling it. Another way to take advantage of the aromatic effect on an appetite is to eat your meal hot (when more odor molecules escape from food) and to smell your food before you eat it. It takes about 20 minutes for your brain to receive the signal that you're full — so gulping food down too quickly can lead to overeating. Here's how to avoid that: take smaller bites of food. When you take smaller bites of something, you end up eating less at a meal because it gives your body the time it needs to digest each bite. Also, set your silverware down between bites. This slows you down to avoid gulping down every forkful. And lastly, chew slowly to savor the flavor and texture.

Realize that food is necessary for survival, but a meal should be enjoyed, not scarfed down. Smell before you eat and take your time eating.

"Small changes can make a big difference."

Unknown-Internet

---

91. Beans, Beans, Good for Your Heart

People who eat beans at least four times a week have a 19% lower risk for heart disease than those who eat beans only once a week (Tulane University study). Do your heart a favor by enjoying more beans. Feast on black bean soup for dinner and you'll help your heart even more. The high amounts of fiber (15 grams per cup —more than half of your daily requirement) and protein (16 grams per cup) in these mostly fat-free powerhouses are responsible for the heart healthy help. You can eat red, kidney or pinto beans as a snack or you can mix them into your favorite rice, salad or soup dish. Next time you're searching for a meal or a snack, remember that beans are filling, tasty, mostly fat-free, and good for your heart.

> *"If we are creating ourselves all the time, then it is never too late to begin creating the bodies we want instead of the ones we mistakenly assume we are stuck with."*
>
> Deepak Chopra

92. Start an Exercise Program at Work

Starting an exercise program at work can include anything from appointing a fitness instructor to teach in an empty conference room, to using a corporate gym for an after-work fitness session. Have a brainstorming session with the coworkers you know who also want to get into shape. Sit down with them over lunch (salads and sparkling water, of course) and come up with as many ideas for the program as you can: What the guidelines could be? If there will be a prize for most weight loss, most committed etc.? How long the program should run? Your program should be at least eight weeks long if anyone wants to see any results; twelve weeks would be better.

At least eight hours a day are spent at your place of business, so why not get a fit body along with your salary? Your co-workers can be used as motivators for maintaining good health while heightening employee morale with a little friendly competition. If your company does not have room for on-site exercise classes, you can still start a healthy exercise program by walking or jogging together before or after work.

> *"You don't always get what you wish for, you get what you work for!"*
>
> *Unknown-Internet*

93. Get a Massage

Massage therapy is an invitation to reconnect with your body. It provides relief from common aches and pains that result from time spent hunched over computers, sitting at desks, or standing for too long. Massage therapy enhances your life by reducing stress, improving circulation and flushing out toxins, while boosting your immune system. A body massage can be soothing, stimulating and invigorating as it releases tension and stress. A full body massage is excellent for relieving tired, aching, knotted muscles that have built up within the system. For you, this means an opportunity to feel truly comfortable in your own body. It is a good, overall relaxing treatment that has the benefits of relieving stiff, sore joints and can be modified to suit the needs of the individual person.

> *"Either you run the day or the day runs you."*
>
> Jim Rohn

94. Surround Yourself with Positive People

The company you keep affects you more than you think. Whether you realize it or not, people's attitudes, perspectives and even their overall moods can rub off on you. This is why it is smart to choose carefully what type of people you're around on a regular basis. You want to associate yourself with positive people — people who want to see you reach new levels of improvement, and who have your best interest at heart. You need people around who will give you the encouragement you need to stay positive when you're feeling less motivated than usual. Surrounding yourself with the right people isn't always as simple as we'd like it to be, but once you get the hang of it, you will start filtering the wrong people out and attracting the right people naturally. Start with yourself! When you exude a positive attitude, smile often, and look at the bright side of almost everything, similar people will naturally be drawn to you and encourage your positive behavior. The more you encourage each other, the more you can expect to benefit mentally and physically.

> *"Surround yourself with people who make you happy. People who make you laugh, who help you when you're in need. People who genuinely care. They are the ones worth keeping in your life. Everyone else is just passing through."*
>
> *Karl Marx*

95. <u>Juice Your Fruits and Vegetables</u>

Juicing your fruits and vegetables is gaining in popularity as more and more people realize that it's a fast and easy way to get the recommended five daily servings of produce in a single glass. Exercise legend Jack Lalanne (the original juicer for the past seven decades) said that, "If you put raw and vital foods in your body, you're going to feel alive and vital." You can juice your fruit and vegetables separately, or you can add fruit to your vegetable blend for a more delightful taste. My preference is to add apple or pineapple to my "green juice" which consists of collard and kale greens, celery, and cucumbers. If you are a juicing virgin you may not want to go out and invest in a juicer just yet. Fortunately, juicing bars are popping up everywhere, so go online and find the closest one near you.

> *"Nothing will benefit human health and increase the chances for survival on earth as much as the evolution to a vegetarian diet."*
>
> *Albert Einstein*

96. Manage and Prevent Diabetes II

Diabetes is a chronic disease that is characterized by the inability of the body to control blood sugar levels. Type II diabetes is a metabolic disorder resulting in too little insulin or lack of proper use of insulin. Lifestyle behaviors and decisions affect the development of type II diabetes. Exercising helps to prevent diabetes II by maintaining insulin's ability to control blood sugar; this is why including physical activity in your life is so important. It's easy to focus on the external benefits of exercise — that's what we're confronted with on a daily basis, but what exercise does for the internal is even more important. Remember, it is permanent weight loss that will make you healthier and lower your diabetes risk. By making small changes, like being more active and eating better, you can alter your lifestyle positively on the outside and inside.

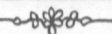

> **"Money is the most envied, but the last enjoyed. Health is the most enjoyed, but last envied"**
>
> *Charles Calebcolton*

97. <u>You Must Commit</u>

If you truly want to create and sustain positive changes in your lifestyle, you must make the decision to fully commit. In order to shed pounds through diet or exercise, consistency is the key. It's been well established that regular exercise performed daily for weeks, and then months, is critical to losing weight. That, plus dietary change, which for most people means cutting fat and limiting portions, is the way to success. These decisions should be paired with your holding yourself accountable for your actions. You must commit to maintaining good health just as you commit to your career, daily responsibilities, relationships and material possessions. If you put time aside each day to exercise and focus on your nutrient intake, you will develop the daily boost and endurance that will stick with you for a lifetime. Unfortunately, most people don't realize how important their health is until it is seriously jeopardized. You don't have to go overboard, but you must commit to a healthy lifestyle in order to see the positive changes associated with it. Don't be afraid to make big goals because success comes from chasing those goals.

> *"Commitment means staying loyal to what you said you were going to do long after the mood you said it in has left you."*
>
> Unknown-Internet

98. Practice Moderation

You've likely heard, and possibly said, one or more of these statements: "I'm on a diet," "I can't have that," "That is not good for me," or, "I was bad today." In an attempt to eat healthier, many of us view certain foods as "bad" or "off limits." This mentality can actually work against efforts toward a healthy lifestyle. Instead of viewing some foods as bad, try focusing on a diet that allows for a variety of foods to be eaten in moderation. An important thing to remember when trying to cut back on empty carbohydrates (food that supplies energy but little or no other nutrition, like cakes, donuts, white rice, fruit flavored beverages) is that it's all about moderation. Foods such as fruits, vegetables and whole grains, should be eaten every day, while fried foods and high in fat snacks should be viewed as occasional treats.

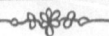

"Eating well is not just about weight loss, it's also about improving your health."

Unknown-Internet

99. <u>Meditate</u>

Meditation requires no special knowledge or background. It's just a personal way to help you unclutter your mind, tune out the world, and temporarily remove any internal and external sources of stress. The practice of meditation can be as simple as closing your eyes and sitting in silence for five minutes during your lunch break. Meditation requires no special location, time of day, or accessories. All you need is a peaceful moment. When you meditate, you become the observer rather than the thinker. Regular practice of this quiet awareness will carry over into your daily life, encouraging physical and emotional balance regardless of what you're confronted with.

"When you expect success, your mind focuses on success."

Unknown-Internet

100. <u>Manage Osteoporosis with Exercise and a Healthy Diet</u>

Consistent exercise and a healthy diet is an effective and inexpensive way to prevent and treat osteoporosis. Osteoporosis is a condition in which the bones become dangerously thin and fragile over time. Exercise works for osteoporosis prevention because it places stress on bones, which builds bone mass. This is especially true for weight bearing and weight training types of exercises. Calcium, the major component of bones, is not well absorbed unless a demand for it is created through exercise. And calcium can be best absorbed by consuming more milk, yogurt, and calcium-fortified orange juice. An estimated 10 million Americans over age 50 have osteoporosis, and another 34 million are at risk. Women account for about 80% of osteoporosis cases, according to Core Concepts In Health, 2013. Don't become a statistic. Strengthen your bones with exercise.

"Workouts are like brushing my teeth; I don't think about them, I just do them. The decision has already been made."

Patti Sue Plumer

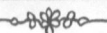

101. <u>Live a Life Filled with Vitality</u>

Some traditional practices for living a long and productive life include not smoking, eating a balanced diet, and maintaining a healthy weight. Beyond the simple presence or absence of disease, overall wellness refers to having optimal health and a vitality for life. This is largely determined by the decisions you make about how you live. So powerful are certain lifestyle choices, that recommended diets, along with maintenance of physical activity and appropriate body mass, can over time reduce the incidence of cancer by thirty to forty percent (American Institute for Cancer Research). Quality of life is equally as important as quantity, which is why so many of the things that can improve longevity can also improve an individual's vitality. Don't just try to live a long life, try to live an amazing one.

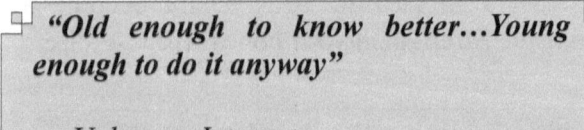

"Old enough to know better...Young enough to do it anyway"

Unknown-Internet

EPILOGUE

Okay, now that you have finished reading *101 Ways to Stay Motivated and Lose Weight*, you may or may not know where to begin. The reading of this book was just step one. Now you are ready to choose one exercise, one diet and one motivational tip to execute or heighten for the next three months. Or maybe you'd rather focus on only one new tip for the next 30 days. Whatever your strategy, I guarantee that as you practice healthy life changing habits, you will become more sensitive and committed to the areas where you desire growth.

My tips are categorized into three groups with an easy to follow table of contents for each (see Categorized Table of Contents in Appendix A).

DIET

If you want to focus on a healthier diet, travel to the Diet section of the Categorized Table of Contents and choose the tip that will most inspire you. You can begin by reducing your portion sizes (#42), eating more fruits and vegetables (#75), and drinking more water (#4). Eating several mini-meals throughout the day also helps you to stay more satisfied as it reduces your hunger at regular mealtime(#15) and family meals.

EXERCISE

My exercise tips are designed to get you moving while explaining the benefits of being physically fit outside of just losing weight. Exercise can lower blood pressure (#84), improve your overall health (#38), and enhance your relationships with your loved ones (#30). Simultaneously, exercise can help you to sleep better (#69), relieve menopause symptoms (#12), and avoid osteoporosis (#100). Regular exercise helps you burn calories faster, even while you're sitting or sleeping, and is generally the best way to maintain weight loss (#7). If you haven't been exercising, but are ready to start consult with your physician first, and schedule a physical examination (#81).

MOTIVATION

Before beginning this process, you must be in the proper frame of mind, as it demands a certain level of commitment (#97), a good bit of aggressiveness (#55), and a realistic attitude (#24). If you have failed at other approaches, take a short time off and gather your thoughts. The key is to learn from your mistakes and to never accept not trying (#18)! Be assured that any sincere effort you put into this endeavor will not be in vain (#48) and know that whenever you try to improve your life, you will always be met with results.

CATEGORIZED TABLE
OF CONTENTS

85. Prepare Healthy Meals with Your Family
87. Beware of Impulsive Vending Machine Snacking
88. Become a Picky Eater
90. Smell Before You Eat and Eat Slowly
91. Beans, Beans, Good for Your Heart
95. Juice Your Fruits and Vegetables

> *"Tell me what you eat, and I will tell you who you are."*
>
> Brillat Savarin

EXERCISE

5. Walk Your Way to Great Health During Lunch
6. Exercise to Help Reduce Low Back Pain
7. Exercise 3-4 Days Per Week
12. Exercise for Menopause Symptom Relief
17. Pick a Time to Exercise and Stick with It
21. Get the Entire Family Involved
26. Join an Aerobics Class
29. "X" Your Calendar When You Exercise
30. Exercise with Your Significant Other
32. Exercise While Watching Television
34. Hire a Personal Trainer
38. Improve Your Overall Health
47. Join a Health Club
51. Run for a Cause
53. Ask for Gifts that Keep on Slimming
54. Add Muscle Toning to Your Workout Routine

> *"We are under-exercised as a nation. We look instead of play. We ride instead of walk. Our existence deprives us of the minimum of physical activity essential for healthy living."*
>
> *President John F. Kennedy*

MOTIVATION

93. Get a Massage
94. Surround Yourself with Positive People
96. Manage and Prevent Diabetes II
97. You Must Commit
98. Practice Moderation
99. Meditate
101. Live a Life Filled with Vitality

> *"Whatever task that you undertake, do it with all your heart and soul. Always be courteous, never be discouraged. Beware of him who promises something for nothing. Do not blame anybody for your mistakes and failures. Do not look for approval except in the consciousness of doing your best."*
>
> *Bernard M. Baruch*

PHYSICAL ACTIVITY HISTORY QUESTIONNAIRE

This brief questionnaire focuses on your current and past experiences with physical activity and the types of things that hindered your progress in the past. The information from this questionnaire can be useful if you are honest about your physical activity history. This allows you to plan for your future without repeating bad choices and re-creating roadblocks from the past.

Physical Activity History Questionnaire

If you **do not** currently participate in physical activity, answer this question:

1. How long has it been since you were physically active or exercised on a regular basis?
   a. Less than 6 months
   b. 6 months to a year
   c. 1 year to 2 years
   d. 2 years to 5 years
   e. 5 years to 10 years
   f. More than 10 years
   g. I have never been physically active or exercised on a consistent basis.

If you **do** currently participate in physical activity, answer the following questions:

1. How many days per week are you physically active?_____
2. Approximately how many minutes are you physically active each day?_____
3. How long have you been physically active at this level?_____
4. What activities do you do regularly?

_____
_____

Answer the following questions whether you **are** currently physically active or **are not** currently physically active.

1. As an adult, were there ever times when you were physically active regularly for at least 3 months and then stopped being physically active for at least 3 months?

    a. Yes   b. No

2. If you answered Yes, how many times did that roadblock occur?_____

3. Regarding the most recent time you hit a roadblock, what specifically halted your progress and caused you to stop being physically active? (Please check all that apply):

____ Lack of money

____ Lack of a facility

____ Lack of a physical activity partner

____ Lack of interest in physical activity

____ Health-related problems

____ Injury

____ Season/weather changes

____ Personal stress

____ Lack of time (due to which of the following, circle any answer that applies): Work or school, household duties, children, social activities, spouse

Other:

_____

The Physical Activity History Questionnaire focuses on your current and past experiences with physical activity and the types of things that got in the way of you continuing with a fitness program in the past. The information from this questionnaire can be useful as you plan your future workouts. To help you jumpover roadblocks from the past, refer back to tip #5, #32, #68, #71, #79 and #92.

SELF-EFFICACY SCALE

This brief, five item Self-Efficacy Scale measures the major components of self-efficacy and has been used in many physical activity studies. If your scores are low, follow some of my tips in this book and complete the questionnaire again in 3 months. As you become more active your scores will increase.

Self-Efficacy Scoring:

Calculate your score for the Self-Efficacy Scale by computing the average of all five items. You must answer all of the items before calculating your score. The higher your average score, the greater your self-efficacy.

Circle the number that indicates how confident you are that you could be physically active in each of the following situations.

SCALE

1 = not at all confident
2 = slightly confident
3 = moderately confident
4 = very confident
5 = extremely confident

1. When I am tired	1	2	3	4	5
2. When I am in a bad mood	1	2	3	4	5
3. When I feel I don't have time	1	2	3	4	5
4. When I am on vacation	1	2	3	4	5
5. When it is raining or snowing	1	2	3	4	5

PHYSICAL ACTIVITY ENJOYMENT SCALE

Many physical activity experts believe that feelings of enjoyment play an important role in helping people continue to be active over time (#46). The Physical Activity Enjoyment Scale is an 18-item measure that can be used to determine how enjoyable exercise is to you. If your score is low, you may want to rethink the type of physical activity you're engaged in and find something that is more enjoyable.

PHYSICAL ACTIVITY
ENJOYMENT SCALE

Please rate how you feel at the moment about physical activity in general. For each feeling, please mark the column that best describes you.

Yes No   Feeling

___ ___ 1. I enjoy it.
___ ___ 2. I like it.
___ ___ 3. I feel bored.
___ ___ 4. I find it pleasureable.
___ ___ 5. I am very absorbed in physical activity.
___ ___ 6. It's a lot of fun.
___ ___ 7. I find it energizing
___ ___ 8. It makes me happy.
___ ___ 9. It's very pleasant.
___ ___ 10. I feel good physically while doing it.
___ ___ 11. It's very invigorating.
___ ___ 12. I am very frustrated by it.
___ ___ 13. It's very gratifying.
___ ___ 14. It's very exhilarating.
___ ___ 15. It's very stimulating.
___ ___ 16. It gives me a strong sense of accomplishment.
___ ___ 17. It's very refreshing
___ ___ 18. I feel as though I would rather be doing something else.

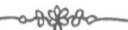

Scoring: **Add up the number of items for which you checked yes. The greater number of yes items, the more likely it is that you enjoy engaging in physical activity.**

ALL ABOUT DONNA

Donna Lynn is an international fitness expert and founder of Donnacize Aerobics, Inc. She is currently a full-time professor of Health & Wellness at Howard University and an adjunct professor at Bowie State University. She's taught classes throughout Luxembourg, Germany, Belgium and France.

For more information about Donna Lynn's products, or to schedule Ms. Lynn to speak or move aerobically with your group, company, association or conference, please call: (443) 600-4895.

Donnacize Aerobics Inc.
donna@donnacize.com
www.donnacize.com